Virtual Clinical Excursion

for

Christensen and Kockrow:
Foundations and Adult Health Nursing
5th Edition

Virtual Clinical Excursions

for

Christensen and Kockrow:
Foundations and Adult Health Nursing
5th Edition

prepared by

Kim D. Cooper, RN, MSN
Ivy Tech Community College
Terre Haute, Indiana

software developed by

Wolfsong Informatics, LLC
Tucson, Arizona

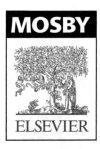

MOSBY

ELSEVIER

11830 Westline Industrial Dr.
St. Louis, Missouri 63146

VIRTUAL CLINICAL EXCURSIONS FOR
CHRISTENSEN AND KOCKROW:
FOUNDATIONS AND ADULT HEALTH NURSING
5TH EDITION
Copyright © 2007 by Mosby, Inc., an affiliate of Elsevier Inc.

ISBN-13: 978-0-323-04339-7
ISBN-10: 0-323-04339-9

Notice

Knowledge and best practice in this field are constantly changing. As new research and experience broaden our knowledge, changes in practice, treatment and drug therapy may become necessary or appropriate. Readers are advised to check the most current information provided (i) on procedures featured or (ii) by the manufacturer of each product to be administered, to verify the recommended dose or formula, the method and duration of administration, and contraindications. It is the responsibility of the practitioner, relying on their own experience and knowledge of the patient, to make diagnoses, to determine dosages and the best treatment for each individual patient, and to take all appropriate safety precautions. To the fullest extent of the law, neither the Publisher nor the Authors assumes any liability for any injury and/or damage to persons or property arising out or related to any use of the material contained in this book.

ISBN-13: 978-0-323-04339-7
ISBN-10: 0-323-04339-9

Executive Editor: *Tom Wilhelm*
Managing Editor: *Jeff Downing*
Associate Developmental Editor: *Tiffany Trautwein*
Project Manager: *Joy Moore*

Printed in the United States of America

Last digit is the print number: 9 8 7 6 5 4

Working together to grow
libraries in developing countries

www.elsevier.com | www.bookaid.org | www.sabre.org

ELSEVIER   BOOK AID International   Sabre Foundation

Workbook
prepared by

Kim D. Cooper, RN, MSN
Ivy Tech Community College
Terre Haute, Indiana

Textbook

Barbara Lauritsen Christensen RN, MS
Nurse Educator
Mid-Plains Community College
North Platte, Nebraska

Elaine Oden Kockrow, RN, MS
Formerly, Nurse Educator
Mid-Plains Community College
North Platte, Nebraska

Contents

Unit 8—Care of the Patient with a Musculoskeletal Disorder

Unit 9—Care of the Surgical Patient

Unit 10—Care of the Patient with a Respiratory Disorder

Unit 11—Care of the Patient with Asthma

Unit 12—Care of the Patient Diagnosed with Cancer

Unit 13—Care of the Patient with a Gastrointestinal Disorder

Table of Contents
Christensen:
Foundations and Adult Health Nursing, 5th Edition

Getting Started

GETTING SET UP

■ **MINIMUM SYSTEM REQUIREMENTS**

WINDOWS®

Windows Vista™, XP, 2000 (Recommend Windows XP/2000)
Pentium® III processor (or equivalent) @ 600 MHz (Recommend 800 MHz or better)
256 MB of RAM (Recommend 1 GB or more for Windows Vista)
800 x 600 screen size (Recommend 1024 x 768)
Thousands of colors
12x CD-ROM drive
Soundblaster 16 soundcard compatibility
Stereo speakers or headphones

Note: Windows Vista and XP require administrator privileges for installation.

MACINTOSH®

MAC OS X (10.2 or higher)
Apple Power PC G3 @ 500 MHz or better
128 MB of RAM (Recommend 256 MB or more)
800 x 600 screen size (Recommend 1024 x 768)
Thousands of colors
12x CD-ROM drive
Stereo speakers or headphones

■ INSTALLATION INSTRUCTIONS

WINDOWS

1. Insert the *Virtual Clinical Excursions—Skilled Nursing* CD-ROM (Disk 1).
2. The setup screen should appear automatically if the current product is not already installed. Windows Vista users may be asked to authorize additional security prompts.
3. Follow the onscreen instructions during the setup process.

   If the setup screen does *not* appear automatically (and *Virtual Clinical Excursions—Skilled Nursing* has not been installed already):
   a. Click the **My Computer** icon on your desktop or on your Start menu.
   b. Double-click on your CD-ROM drive.
   c. If installation does not start at this point:
      (1) Click the **Start** icon on the taskbar and select the **Run** option.
      (2) Type d:\setup.exe (where "d:\" is your CD-ROM drive) and press **OK**.
      (3) Follow the onscreen instructions for installation.

4. For lessons that require the use of the *Virtual Clinical Excursions—Medical-Surgical* program (Disk 2), repeat the above steps to install that program.

MACINTOSH

1. Insert the *Virtual Clinical Excursions—Skilled Nursing* or *Medical-Surgical* CD in the CD-ROM drive. The disk icon will appear on your desktop.

2. Double-click on the disk icon.

3. Double-click on the VCESN_MAC or MEDICAL-SURGICAL_MAC run file.

Note: Virtual Clinical Excursions—Skilled Nursing and *Medical-Surgical* for Macintosh do not have an installation setup and can only be run directly from the CD.

■ HOW TO USE VIRTUAL CLINICAL EXCURSIONS

WINDOWS

1. Double-click on the *Virtual Clinical Excursions—Skilled Nursing* or *Medical-Surgical* icon located on your desktop.
2. Or navigate to the program via the Windows Start menu.

Note: If your computer uses Windows Vista, right-click on the desktop shortcut and choose **Properties**. In the Compatability Mode, check the box for "Run as Administrator." Below is a screen capture to show what this looks like.

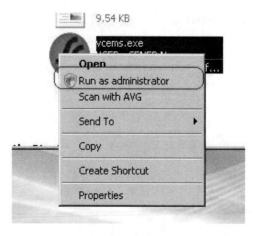

MACINTOSH

1. Insert the *Virtual Clinical Excursions—Skilled Nursing* or *Medical-Surgical* CD in the CD-ROM drive. The disk icon will appear on your desktop.

2. Double-click on the disk icon.

3. Double-click on the VCESN_MAC or MEDICAL-SURGICAL_MAC run file.

Note: Virtual Clinical Excursions—Skilled Nursing or *Medical-Surgical* for Macintosh do not have an installation setup and can only be run directly from the CD.

■ SCREEN SETTINGS

For best results, your computer monitor resolution should be set at a minimum of 800 x 600. The number of colors displayed should be set to "thousands or higher" (High Color or 16 bit) or "millions of colors" (True Color or 24 bit).

Windows

1. From the **Start** menu, select **Control Panel** (on some systems, you will first go to **Settings**, then to **Control Panel**).
2. Double-click on the **Display** icon.
3. Click on the **Settings** tab.
4. Under **Screen resolution** use the slider bar to select **800 by 600 pixels**.
5. Access the **Colors** drop-down menu by clicking on the down arrow.
6. Select **High Color (16 bit)** or **True Color (24 bit)**.
7. Click on **OK**.
8. You may be asked to verify the setting changes. Click **Yes**.
9. You may be asked to restart your computer to accept the changes. Click **Yes**.

Macintosh

1. Select the **Monitors** control panel.
2. Select **800 x 600** (or similar) from the **Resolution** area.
3. Select **Thousands** or **Millions** from the **Color Depth** area.

■ WEB BROWSERS

Supported web browsers include Microsoft Internet Explorer (IE) version 6.0 or higher and Mozilla Firefox version 2.0 or higher. The supported browser for Macs running OS X is Mozilla Firefox.

If you use America Online® (AOL) for web access, you will need AOL version 4.0 or higher and one of the browsers listed above. Do not use earlier versions of AOL with earlier versions of IE, because you will have difficulty accessing many features.

For best results with AOL:
*   Connect to the Internet using AOL version 4.0 or higher.
*   Open a private chat within AOL (this allows the AOL client to remain open, without asking whether you wish to disconnect while minimized).
*   Minimize AOL.
*   Launch a recommended browser.

■ **TECHNICAL SUPPORT**

Technical support for this product is available between 7:30 a.m. and 7 p.m. (CST), Monday through Friday. Before calling, be sure that your computer meets the minimum system requirements to run this software. Inside the United States and Canada, call 1-800-692-9010. Outside North America, call 314-872-8370. You may also fax your questions to 314-523-4932 or contact Technical Support through e-mail: technical.support@elsevier.com.

Trademarks: Windows, Macintosh, Pentium, and America Online are registered trademarks.

ACCESSING *Virtual Clinical Excursions* FROM EVOLVE

The product you have purchased is part of the Evolve family of online courses and learning resources. Please read the following information thoroughly to get started.

To access your instructor's course on Evolve:

Your instructor will provide you with the username and password needed to access this specific course on the Evolve Learning System. Once you have received this information, please follow these instructions:

1. Go to the Evolve student page (http://evolve.elsevier.com/student).

2. Enter your username and password in the **Login to My Evolve** area and click the **Login** button.

3. You will be taken to your personalized **My Evolve** page, where the course will be listed in the **My Courses** module.

TECHNICAL REQUIREMENTS

To use an Evolve course, you will need access to a computer that is connected to the Internet and equipped with web browser software that supports frames. For optimal performance, it is recommended that you have speakers and use a high-speed Internet connection. However, slower dial-up modems (56 K minimum) are acceptable.

Whichever browser you use, the browser preferences must be set to enable cookies and JavaScript and the cache must be set to reload every time.

Enable Cookies

Browser	Steps
Internet Explorer (IE) 6.0 or higher	1. Select **Tools → Internet Options**. 2. Select **Privacy** tab. 3. Use the slider (slide down) to **Accept All Cookies**. 4. Click **OK**. -OR- 3. Click the **Advanced** button. 4. Click the check box next to **Override Automatic Cookie Handling**. 5. Click the **Accept** radio buttons under **First-party Cookies** and **Third-party Cookies**. 6. Click **OK**.
Mozilla Firefox 2.0 or higher	1. Select **Tools → Options**. 2. Select the **Privacy** icon. 3. Click to expand Cookies. 4. Select **Allow sites to set cookies**. 5. Click **OK**.

Set Cache to Always Reload a Page

Browser	Steps
Internet Explorer (IE) 6.0 or higher	1. Select **Tools → Internet Options**. 2. Select **General** tab. 3. Go to the **Temporary Internet Files** and click the **Settings** button. 4. Select the radio button for **Every visit to the page** and click **OK** when complete.
Mozilla Firefox 2.0 or higher	1. Select **Tools → Options**. 2. Select the **Privacy** icon. 3. Click to expand Cache. 4. Set the value to "0" in the **Use up to: __ MB of disk space for the cache** field. 5. Click **OK**.

Plug-Ins

Adobe Acrobat Reader—With the free Acrobat Reader software, you can view and print Adobe PDF files. Many Evolve products offer student and instructor manuals, checklists, and more in this format!

Download at: http://www.adobe.com

Apple QuickTime—Install this to hear word pronunciations, heart and lung sounds, and many other helpful audio clips within Evolve Online Courses!

Download at: http://www.apple.com

Adobe Flash Player—This player will enhance your viewing of many Evolve web pages, as well as educational short-form to long-form animation within the Evolve Learning System!

Download at: http://www.adobe.com

Adobe Shockwave Player—Shockwave is best for viewing the many interactive learning activities within Evolve Online Courses!

Download at: http://www.adobe.com

Microsoft Word Viewer—With this viewer, Microsoft Word users can share documents with those who don't have Word, and users without Word can open and view Word documents. Many Evolve products have testbank, student and instructor manuals, and other documents available for downloading and viewing on your own computer!

Download at: http://www.microsoft.com

Microsoft PowerPoint Viewer—With this viewer, you can access PowerPoint 97, 2000, and 2002 presentations even if you don't have PowerPoint. Many Evolve products have slides available for downloading and viewing on your own computer!

Download at: http://www.microsoft.com

SUPPORT INFORMATION

Live phone support is available to customers in the United States and Canada at **800-401-9962** from 7:30 a.m. to 7 p.m. (CST), Monday through Friday. Support is also available through email at evolve-support@elsevier.com.

Online 24/7 support can be accessed on the Evolve website (http://evolve.elsevier.com). Resources include:

- Guided tours
- Tutorials
- Frequently asked questions (FAQs)
- Online copies of course user guides
- And much more!

A QUICK TOUR

Welcome to *Virtual Clinical Excursions*, a virtual hospital setting in which you can work with multiple complex patient simulations and also learn to access and evaluate the information resources that are essential for high-quality patient care. The virtual hospital, Pacific View Regional Hospital, has realistic architecture and access to patient rooms, a Nurses' Station, and a Medication Room.

■ BEFORE YOU START

Make sure you have your textbook nearby when you use the *Virtual Clinical Excursions—Skilled Nursing* and *Medical-Surgical* CDs. You will want to consult topic areas in your textbook frequently while working with the CD and using this workbook. At the beginning of each lesson, you will be instructed to use either the *Skilled Nursing* or *Medical-Surgical* CD.

■ HOW TO SIGN IN

- Insert the *Virtual Clinical Excursions—Medical-Surgical* CD (Disk 2).
- Once the program has loaded, enter your name on the Student Nurse identification badge.
- Now choose one of the four periods of care in which to work. In Periods of Care 1 through 3, you can actively engage in patient assessment, entry of data in the electronic patient record (EPR), and medication administration. Period of Care 4 presents the day in review. Highlight and click the appropriate period of care. (For this quick tour, choose **Period of Care 1: 0730-0815**.)
- This takes you to the Patient List screen (see example on page 11). Only the patients on the Medical-Surgical Floor are available. Note that the virtual time is provided in the box at the lower left corner of the screen (0730, since we chose Period of Care 1).

Note: If you choose to work during Period of Care 4: 1900-2000, the Patient List screen is skipped since you are not able to visit patients or administer medications during the shift. Instead, you are taken directly to the Nurses' Station, where the records of all the patients on the floor are available for your review.

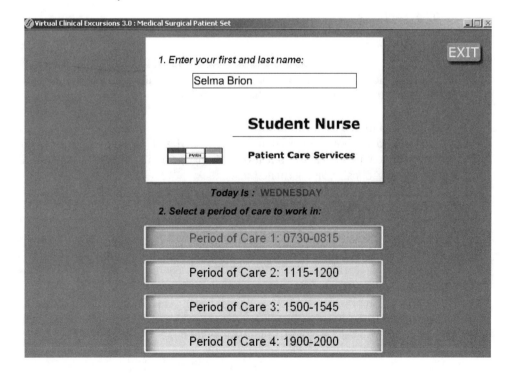

■ **PATIENT LIST (Disk 1)**

SKILLED NURSING UNIT

William Jefferson (Room 501)
Alzheimer's disease—A 75-year-old African-American male admitted for stabilization of type 2 diabetes and hypertension following a recent acute care admission for a urinary tract infection and sepsis. His complications include episodes of acute delirium and a history of osteoarthritis.

Delores Gallegos (Room 502)
Congestive heart failure—An 82-year-old Hispanic female admitted to the Skilled Nursing Unit for congestive heart failure. During her stay it is determined that she has dermatitis, as well as emerging pneumonia.

Kathryn Doyle (Room 503)
Rehabilitation post left hip replacement—A 79-year-old Caucasian female admitted following a complicated recovery from an ORIF. She is experiencing symptoms of malnutrition and depression due to unstable family dynamics, placing her at risk for elder abuse.

Carlos Reyes (Room 504)
Rehabilitation status post myocardial infarction—An 81-year-old Hispanic male admitted for evaluation of the need for long-term care following an acute care hospital stay. Recent cognitive changes and a diagnosis of anxiety disorder contribute to stressful family dynamics and caregiver strain.

Goro Oishi (Room 505)
Hospice care—A 66-year-old Asian male admitted following an acute care admission for an intracerebral hemorrhage and resulting coma. Family-staff interactions provide opportunities to explore death and dying issues related to conflict about advanced life support and cultural and religious differences.

PATIENT LIST (Disk 2)

MEDICAL-SURGICAL UNIT

Harry George (Room 401)
Osteomyelitis—A 54-year-old Caucasian male admitted from a homeless shelter with an infected leg. He has complications of type 2 diabetes mellitus, alcohol abuse, nicotine addiction, poor pain control, and complex psychosocial issues.

Jacquline Catanazaro (Room 402)
Asthma—A 45-year-old Caucasian female admitted with an acute asthma exacerbation and suspected pneumonia. She has complications of chronic schizophrenia, noncompliance with medication therapy, obesity, and herniated disc.

Piya Jordan (Room 403)
Bowel obstruction—A 68-year-old Asian female admitted with a colon mass and suspected adenocarcinoma. She undergoes a right hemicolectomy. This patient's complications include atrial fibrillation, hypokalemia, and symptoms of meperidine toxicity.

Clarence Hughes (Room 404)
Degenerative joint disease—A 73-year-old African-American male admitted for a left total knee replacement. His preparations for discharge are complicated by the development of a pulmonary embolus and the need for ongoing intravenous therapy.

Pablo Rodriguez (Room 405)
Metastatic lung carcinoma—A 71-year-old Hispanic male admitted with symptoms of dehydration and malnutrition. He has chronic pain secondary to multiple subcutaneous skin nodules and psychosocial concerns related to family issues with his approaching death.

Patricia Newman (Room 406)
Pneumonia—A 61-year-old Caucasian female admitted with worsening pulmonary function and an acute respiratory infection. Her chronic emphysema is complicated by heavy smoking, hypertension, and malnutrition. She needs access to community resources such as a smoking cessation program and meal assistance.

■ HOW TO SELECT A PATIENT

- You can choose one or more patients to work with from the Patient List by checking the box to the left of the patient name(s). For this quick tour, select Piya Jordan and Pablo Rodriguez. (In order to receive a scorecard for a patient, the patient must be selected before proceeding to the Nurses' Station.)
- Click on **Get Report** to the right of the medical records number (MRN) to view a summary of the patient's care during the 12-hour period before your arrival on the unit.
- After reviewing the report, click on **Go to Nurses' Station** in the right lower corner to begin your care. (*Note:* If you have been assigned to care for multiple patients, you can click on **Return to Patient List** to select and review the report for each additional patient before going to the Nurses' Station.)

Note: Even though the Patient List is initially skipped when you sign in to work for Period of Care 4, you can still access this screen if you wish to review the shift report for any of the patients. To do so, simply click on **Patient List** near the top left corner of the Nurses' Station (or click on the clipboard to the left of the Kardex). Then click on **Get Report** for the patient(s) whose care you are reviewing. This may be done during any period of care.

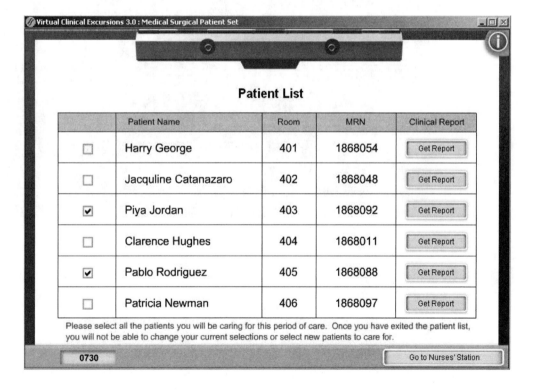

■ HOW TO FIND A PATIENT'S RECORDS

NURSES' STATION

Within the Nurses' Station, you will see:

1. A clipboard that contains the patient list for that floor.
2. A chart rack with patient charts labeled by room number, a notebook labeled Kardex, and a notebook labeled MAR (Medication Administration Record).
3. A desktop computer with access to the Electronic Patient Record (EPR).
4. A tool bar across the top of the screen that can also be used to access the Patient List, EPR, Chart, MAR, and Kardex. This tool bar is also accessible from each patient's room.
5. A Drug Guide containing information about the medications you are able to administer to your patients.
6. A tool bar across the bottom of the screen that can be used to access the Floor Map, patient rooms, Medication Room, and Drug Guide.

As you run your cursor over an item, it will be highlighted. To select, simply double-click on the item. As you use these resources, you will always be able to return to the Nurses' Station by clicking on the **Return to Nurses' Station** bar located in the right lower corner of your screen.

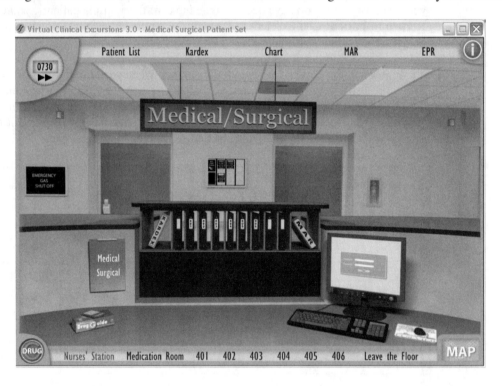

MEDICATION ADMINISTRATION RECORD (MAR)

The MAR icon located on the tool bar at the top of your screen accesses current 24-hour medications for each patient. Click on the icon and the MAR will open. (*Note:* You can also access the MAR by clicking on the MAR notebook on the far right side of the book rack in the center of the screen.) Within the MAR, tabs on the right side of the screen allow you to select patients by room number. Be careful to make sure you select the correct tab number for *your* patient rather than simply reading the first record that appears after the MAR opens. Each MAR sheet lists the following:

- Medications
- Route and dosage of each medication
- Times of administration of each medication

Note: The MAR changes each day. Expired MARs are stored in the patients' charts.

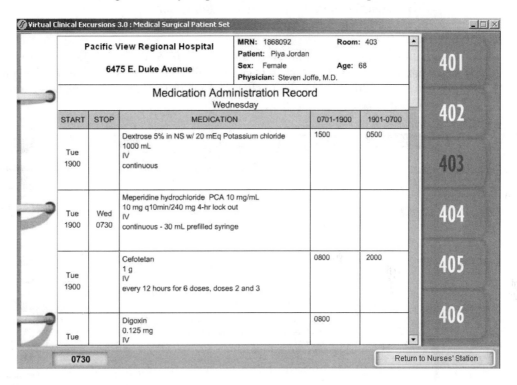

CHARTS

To access patient charts, either click on the **Chart** icon at the top of your screen or anywhere within the chart rack in the center of the Nurses' Station screen. When the close-up view appears, the individual charts are labeled by room number. To open a chart, click on the room number of the patient whose chart you wish to review. The patient's name and allergies will appear on the left side of the screen, along with a list of tabs on the right side of the screen, allowing you to view the following data:

- Allergies
- Physician's Orders
- Physician's Notes
- Nurse's Notes
- Laboratory Reports
- Diagnostic Reports
- Surgical Reports
- Consultations

- Patient Education
- History and Physical
- Nursing Admission
- Expired MARs
- Consents
- Mental Health
- Admissions
- Emergency Department

Information appears in real time. The entries are in reverse chronologic order, so use the down arrow at the right side of each chart page to scroll down to view previous entries. Flip from tab to tab to view multiple data fields or click on **Return to Nurses' Station** in the lower right corner of the screen to exit the chart.

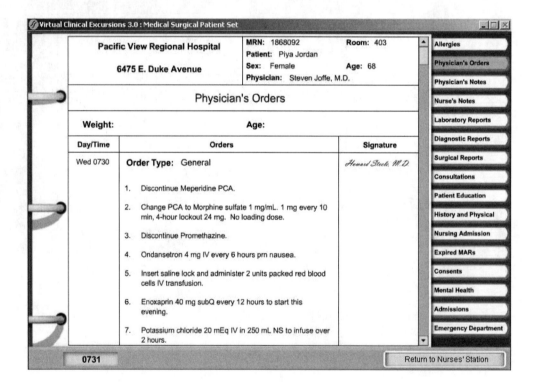

ELECTRONIC PATIENT RECORD (EPR)

The EPR can be accessed from the computer in the Nurses' Station or from the EPR icon located in the tool bar at the top of your screen. To access a patient's EPR:
- Click on either the computer screen or the **EPR** icon.
- Your username and password are automatically filled in.
- Click on **Login** to enter the EPR.
- *Note:* Like the MAR, the EPR is arranged numerically. Thus when you enter, you are initially shown the records of the patient in the lowest room number on the floor. To view the correct data for *your* patient, remember to select the correct room number, using the drop-down menu for the Patient field at the top left corner of the screen.

The EPR used in Pacific View Regional Hospital represents a composite of commercial versions being used in hospitals. You can access the EPR:
- to review existing data for a patient (by room number).
- to enter data you collect while working with a patient.

The EPR is updated daily, so no matter what day or part of a shift you are working, there will be a current EPR with the patient's data from the past days of the current hospital stay. This type of simulated EPR allows you to examine how data for different attributes have changed over time, as well as to examine data for all of a patient's attributes at a particular time. The EPR is fully functional (as it is in a real-life hospital). You can enter such data as blood pressure, breath sounds, and certain treatments. The EPR will not, however, allow you to enter data for a previous time period. Use the arrows at the bottom of the screen to move forward and backward in time.

Virtual Clinical Excursions 3.0 : Medical Surgical Patient Set				_ □ ×
Patient: 403 ▼ **Category:** Vital Signs ▼				**0732**

Name: Piya Jordan	Wed 0630	Wed 0700	Wed 0715	Code Meanings	
PAIN: LOCATION		OS		A	Abdomen
PAIN: RATING		5		Ar	Arm
PAIN: CHARACTERISTICS		C		B	Back
PAIN: VOCAL CUES		VC3		C	Chest
PAIN: FACIAL CUES		FC1		Ft	Foot
PAIN: BODILY CUES				H	Head
PAIN: SYSTEM CUES				Hd	Hand
PAIN: FUNCTIONAL EFFECTS				L	Left
PAIN: PREDISPOSING FACTORS				Lg	Leg
PAIN: RELIEVING FACTORS				Lw	Lower
PCA		P		N	Neck
TEMPERATURE (F)		99.6		NN	See Nurses notes
TEMPERATURE (C)				OS	Operative site
MODE OF MEASUREMENT		Ty		Or	See Physicians orders
SYSTOLIC PRESSURE		110		PN	See Progress notes
DIASTOLIC PRESSURE		70		R	Right
BP MODE OF MEASUREMENT		NIBP		Up	Upper
HEART RATE		104			
RESPIRATORY RATE		18			
SpO2 (%)		95			
BLOOD GLUCOSE					
WEIGHT					
HEIGHT					

◄   ►   Exit EPR

At the top of the EPR screen, you can choose patients by their room numbers. In addition, you have access to 17 different categories of patient data. To change patients or data categories, click the down arrow to the right of the room number or category.

The categories of patient data in the EPR as as follows:

- Vital Signs
- Respiratory
- Cardiovascular
- Neurologic
- Gastrointestinal
- Excretory
- Musculoskeletal
- Integumentary
- Reproductive
- Psychosocial
- Wounds and Drains
- Activity
- Hygiene and Comfort
- Safety
- Nutrition
- IV
- Intake and Output

Remember, each hospital selects its own codes. The codes used in the EPR at Pacific View Regional Hospital may be different from ones you have seen in your clinical rotations. Take some time to acquaint yourself with the codes. Within the Vital Signs category, click on any item in the left column (e.g., Pain: Characteristics). In the far-right column, you will see a list of code meanings for the possible findings and/or descriptors for that assessment area.

You will use the codes to record the data you collect as you work with patients. Click on the box in the last time column to the right of any item and wait for the code meanings applicable to that entry to appear. Select the appropriate code to describe your assessment findings and type it in the box. (*Note:* If no cursor appears within the box, click on the box again until the blue shading disappears and the blinking cursor appears.) Once the data are typed in this box, they are entered into the patient's record for this period of care only.

To leave the EPR, click on **Exit EPR** in the bottom right corner of the screen.

■ VISITING A PATIENT

From the Nurses' Station, click on the room number of the patient you wish to visit (in the tool bar at the bottom of your screen). Once you are inside the room, you will see a still photo of your patient in the top left corner. To verify that this is the correct patient, click on the **Check Armband** icon to the right of the photo. The patient's identification data will appear. If you click on **Check Allergies** (the next icon to the right), a list of the patient's allergies (if any) will replace the photo.

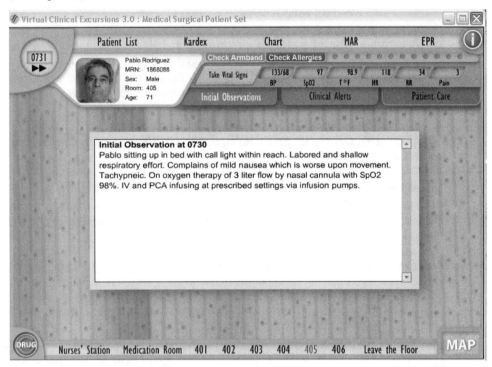

Also located in the patient's room are multiple icons you can use to assess the patient or the patient's medications. A virtual clock is provided in the upper left corner of the room to monitor your progress in real time. (*Note:* The fast-forward icon within the virtual clock will advance the time by 2-minute intervals when clicked.)

- The tool bar across the top of the screen allows you to check the **Patient List**, access the **EPR** to check or enter data, and view the patient's **Chart**, **MAR**, or **Kardex**.
- The **Take Vital Signs** icon allows you to measure the patient's up-to-the-minute blood pressure, oxygen saturation, temperature, heart rate, respiratory rate, and pain level.
- Each time you enter a patient's room, you are given an Initial Observation report to review (in the text box under the patient's photo). These notes are provided to give you a "look" at the patient as if you had just stepped into the room. You can also click on the **Initial Observations** icon to return to this box from other views within the patient's room. To the right of this icon is **Clinical Alerts**, a resource that allows you to make decisions about priority medication interventions based on emerging data collected in real time. Check this screen throughout your period of care to avoid missing critical information related to recently ordered or STAT medications.
- Clicking on **Patient Care** opens up three specific learning environments within the patient room: **Physical Assessment**, **Nurse-Client Interactions**, and **Medication Administration**.
- To perform a **Physical Assessment**, choose a body area (such as **Head & Neck**) from the column of yellow buttons. This activates a list of system subcategories for that body area (e.g., see **Sensory**, **Neurologic**, etc. in the green boxes). After you select the system you wish to evaluate, a brief description of the assessment findings will appear in a box to the right. A still photo provides a "snapshot" of how an assessment of this area might be done or what the finding might look like. For every body area, you can also click on **Equipment** on the right side of the screen.

- To the right of the Physical Assessment icon is **Nurse-Client Interactions**. Clicking on this icon will reveal the times and titles of any videos available for viewing. (*Note:* If the video you wish to see is not listed, this means you have not yet reached the correct virtual time to view that video. Check the virtual clock; you may return to access the video once its designated time has occurred—as long as you do so within the same period of care. Or you can click on the fast-forward icon within the virtual clock to advance the time by 2-minute intervals. You will then need to click again on **Patient Care** and **Nurse-Client Interactions** to refresh the screen.) To view a listed video, click on the white arrow to the right of the video title. Use the control buttons below the video to start, stop, pause, rewind, or fast-forward the action or to mute the sound.
- **Medication Administration** is the pathway that allows you to review and administer medications to a patient after you have prepared them in the Medication Room. This process is addressed further in the *How to Prepare Medications* section (pages 19-20) and in *Medications* (pages 26-30). For additional hands-on practice, see *Reducing Medication Errors* (pages 37-41).

■ HOW TO QUIT, CHANGE PATIENTS, CHANGE PERIOD OF CARE, OR CHANGE DISKS

How to Quit: From most screens, you may click the **Leave the Floor** icon on the bottom tool bar to the right of the patient room numbers. (*Note:* From some screens, you will first need to click an **Exit** button or **Return to Nurses' Station** before clicking **Leave the Floor**.) When the Floor Menu appears, click **Exit** to leave the program.

How to Change Patients or Periods of Care: To change patients, simply click on the new patient's room number. (You cannot receive a scorecard for a new patient, however, unless you have already selected that patient on the Patient List screen.) To change to a new period of care or to restart the virtual clock, click on **Leave the Floor** and then on **Restart the Program**.

How to Change Disks: The lessons in this workbook use two different VCE CDs—one for patients on Floor 5, Skilled Nursing (Disk 1) and one for patients on Floor 4, Medical-Surgical (Disk 2). To select a patient on a different floor, click **Exit the Program** and then click the desktop icon for the other disk.

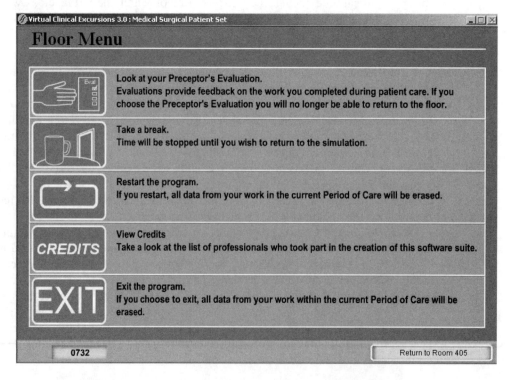

■ HOW TO PREPARE MEDICATIONS

From the Nurses' Station or the patient's room, you can access the Medication Room by clicking on the icon in the tool bar at the bottom of your screen to the left of the patient room numbers.

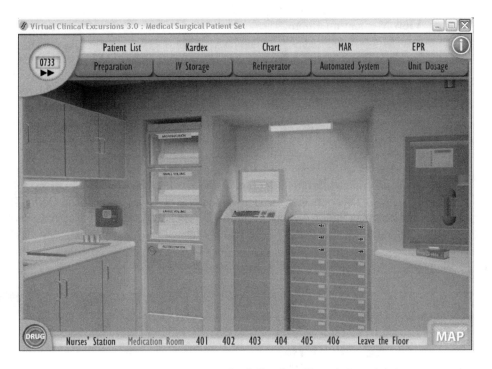

In the Medication Room you have access to the following (from left to right):

- A preparation area is located on the counter under the cabinets. To begin the medication preparation process, click on the tray on the counter or click on the **Preparation** icon at the top of the screen. The next screen leads you through a specific sequence (called the Preparation Wizard) to prepare medications one at a time for administration to a patient. However, no medication has been selected at this time. We will do this while working with a patient in *A Detailed Tour*. To exit this screen, click on **View Medication Room**.

- To the right of the cabinets (and above the refrigerator), IV storage bins are provided. Click on the bins themselves or on the **IV Storage** icon at the top of the screen. The bins are labeled **Microinfusion**, **Small Volume**, and **Large Volume**. Click on an individual bin to see a list of its contents. If you needed to prepare an IV medication at this time, you could click on the medication and its label would appear to the right under the patient's name. (*Note:* You can **Open** and **Close** any medication label by clicking the appropriate icon.) Next, you would click **Put Medication on Tray**. If you ever change your mind or decide that you have put the incorrect medication on the tray, you can reverse your actions by highlighting the medication on the tray and then clicking **Put Medication in Bin**. Click **Close Bin** in the right bottom corner to exit. **View Medication Room** brings you back to a full view of the entire room.

- A refrigerator is located under the IV storage bins to hold any medications that must be stored below room temperature. Click on the refrigerator door or on the **Refrigerator** icon at the top of the screen. Then click on the close-up view of the door to access the medications. When you are finished, click **Close Door** and then **View Medication Room**.

- To prepare controlled substances, click the **Automated System** icon at the top of the screen or click the computer monitor located to the right of the IV storage bins. A login screen will appear; your name and password are automatically filled in. Click **Login**. Select the patient for whom you wish to access medications; then select the correct medication drawer to open (they are stored alphabetically). Click **Open Drawer**, highlight the proper medication, and choose **Put Medication on Tray**. When you are finished, click **Close Drawer** and then **View Medication Room**.

- Next to the Automated System is a set of drawers identified by patient room number. To access these, click on the drawers or on the **Unit Dosage** icon at the top of the screen. This provides a close-up view of the drawers. To open a drawer, click on the room number of the patient you are working with. Next, click on the medication you would like to prepare for the patient, and a label will appear, listing the medication strength, units, and dosage per unit. To exit, click **Close Drawer**; then click **View Medication Room**.

At any time, you can learn about a medication you wish to prepare for a patient by clicking on the **Drug** icon in the bottom left corner of the medication room screen or by clicking the **Drug Guide** book on the counter to the right of the unit dosage drawers. The **Drug Guide** provides information about the medications commonly included in nursing drug handbooks. Nutritional supplements and maintenance intravenous fluid preparations are not included. Highlight a medication in the alphabetical list; relevant information about the drug will appear in the screen below. To exit, click **Return to Medication Room**.

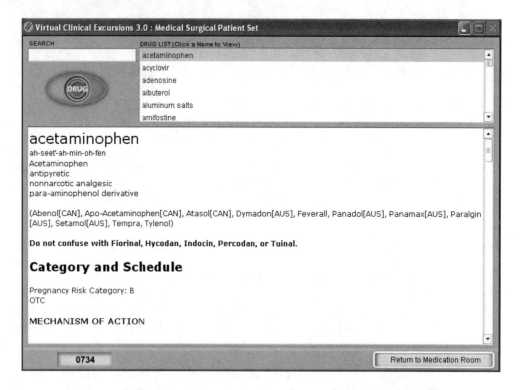

To access the MAR to review the medications ordered for a patient, click on the **MAR** icon located in the tool bar at the top of your screen and then click on the correct tab for your patient's room number. You may also click the **Review MAR** icon in the tool bar at the bottom of your screen from inside each medication storage area.

After you have chosen and prepared medications, go to the patient's room to administer them by clicking on the room number in the bottom tool bar. Inside the patient's room, click **Patient Care** and then **Medication Administration** and follow the proper administration sequence.

■ PRECEPTOR'S EVALUATIONS

When you have finished a session, click on **Leave the Floor** to go to the Floor Menu. At this point, you can click on the top icon (**Look at Your Preceptor's Evaluation**) to receive a score-card that provides feedback on the work you completed during patient care.

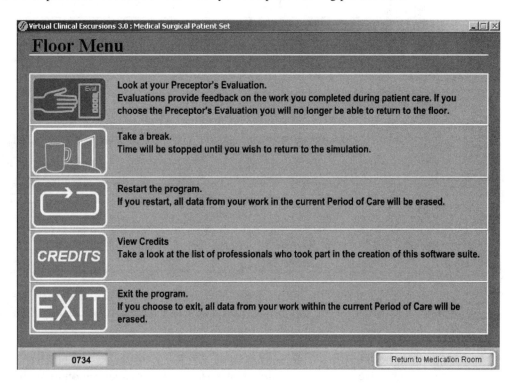

Evaluations are available for each patient you selected when you signed in for the current period of care. Click on the **Medication Scorecard** icon to see an example.

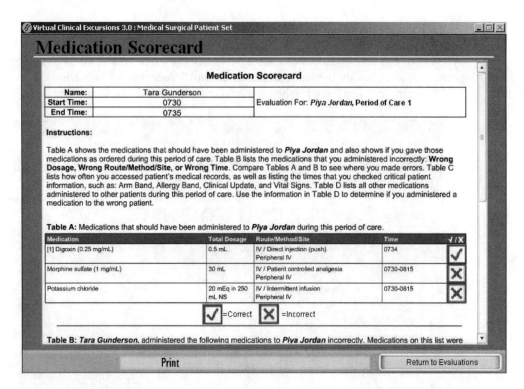

The scorecard compares the medications you administered to a patient during a period of care with what should have been administered. Table A lists the correct medications. Table B lists any medications that were administered incorrectly.

Remember, not every medication listed on the MAR should necessarily be given. For example, a patient might have an allergy to a drug that was ordered, or a medication might have been improperly transcribed to the MAR. Predetermined medication "errors" embedded within the program challenge you to exercise critical thinking skills and professional judgment when deciding to administer a medication, just as you would in a real hospital. Use all your available resources, such as the patient's chart and the MAR, to make your decision.

Table C lists the resources that were available to assist you in medication administration. It also documents whether and when you accessed these resources. For example, did you check the patient armband or perform a check of vital signs? If so, when?

You can click **Print** to get a copy of this report if needed. When you have finished reviewing the scorecard, click **Return to Evaluations** and then **Return to Menu**.

■ FLOOR MAP

To get a general sense of your location within the hospital, you can click on the **Map** icon found in the lower right corner of most of the screens in the *Virtual Clinical Excursions—Skilled Nursing* or *Medical-Surgical* program. (*Note:* If you are following this quick tour step by step, you will need to **Restart the Program** from the Floor Menu, sign in again, and go to the Nurses' Station to access the map.) When you click the **Map** icon, a floor map appears, showing the layout of the floor you are currently on, as well as a directory of the patients and services on that floor. As you move your cursor over the directory list, the location of each room is highlighted on the map (and vice versa). The floor map can be accessed from the Nurses' Station, Medication Room, and each patient's room.

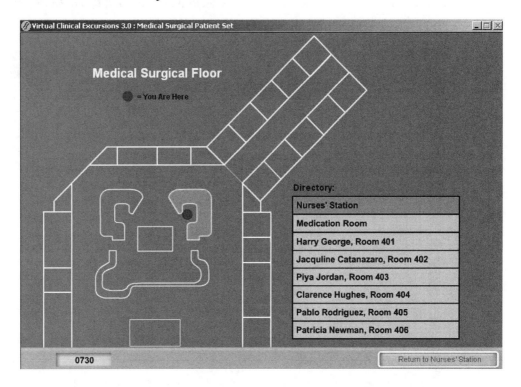

A DETAILED TOUR

If you wish to more thoroughly understand the capabilities of *Virtual Clinical Excursions*, take a detailed tour by completing the following section. During this tour, we will work with a specific patient to introduce you to all the different components and learning opportunities available within the software.

■ WORKING WITH A PATIENT

Using the *Virtual Clinical Excursions—Medical-Surgical* CD (Disk 2), sign in for Period of Care 1 (0730-0815). From the Patient List, select Piya Jordan and Pablo Rodriguez; however, do not go to the Nurses' Station yet.

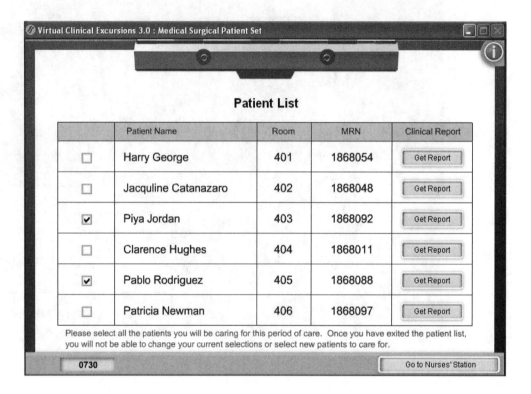

■ REPORT

In hospitals, when one shift ends and another begins, the outgoing nurse who attended a patient will give a verbal and sometimes a written summary of that patient's condition to the incoming nurse who will assume care for the patient. This summary is called a report and is an important source of data to provide an overview of a patient. Your first task is to get the clinical report on Piya Jordan. To do this, click **Get Report** in the far right column in this patient's row. From a brief review of this summary, identify the problems and areas of concern that you will need to address for this patient.

When you have finished noting any areas of concern, click **Go to Nurses' Station**.

■ CHARTS

You can access Piya Jordan's chart from the Nurses' Station or from the patient's room (403). From the Nurses' Station, click on the chart rack or on the **Chart** icon in the tool bar at the top of your screen. Next, click on the chart labeled **403** to open the medical record for Piya Jordan. Click on the **Emergency Department** tab to view a record of why this patient was admitted.

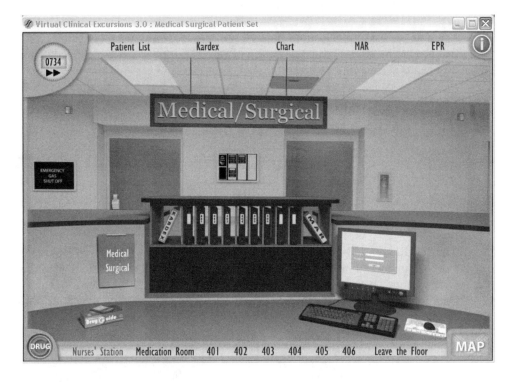

How many days has Piya Jordan been in the hospital?

What tests were done upon her arrival in the Emergency Department and why?

What was her reason for admission?

You should also click on **Surgical Reports** to learn what procedures were performed and when. Finally, review the **Nursing Admission** and **History and Physical** to learn about the health history of this patient. When you are done reviewing the chart, click **Return to Nurses' Station**.

■ MEDICATIONS

Open the Medication Administration Record (MAR) by clicking on the **MAR** icon in the tool bar at the top of your screen. *Remember:* The MAR automatically opens to the first occupied room number on the floor—which is not necessarily your patient's room number! Since you need to access Piya Jordan's MAR, click on tab **403** (her room number). Always make sure you are giving the *Right Drug to the Right Patient!*

Examine the list of medications ordered for Piya Jordan. In the table below, list the medications that need to be given during this period of care (0730-0815). For each medication, note the dosage, route, and time to be given.

Time	Medication	Dosage	Route

Click on **Return to Nurses' Station**. Next, click on **403** on the bottom tool bar and then verify that you are indeed in Piya Jordan's room. Select **Clinical Alerts** (the icon to the right of Initial Observations) to check for any emerging data that might affect your medication administration priorities. Next, go to the patient's chart (click on the **Chart** icon; then click on **403**). When the chart opens, select the **Physician's Orders** tab.

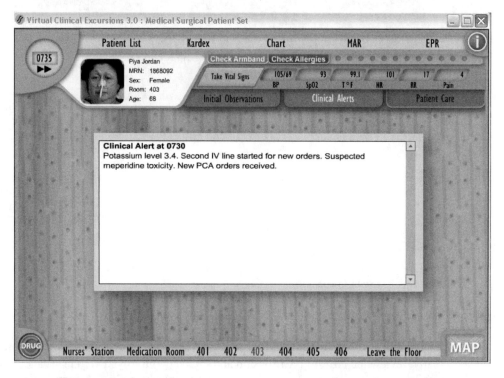

Review the orders. Have any new medications been ordered? Return to the MAR (click **Return to Room 403**; then click **MAR**). Verify that the new medications have been correctly transcribed to the MAR. Mistakes are sometimes made in the transcription process in the hospital setting, and it is sound practice to double-check any new order.

Are there any patient assessments you will need to perform before administering these medications? If so, return to Room 403 and click on **Patient Care** and then **Physical Assessment** to complete those assessments before proceeding.

Now click on the **Medication Room** icon in the tool bar at the bottom of your screen to locate and prepare the medications for Piya Jordan.

In the Medication Room, you must access the medications for Piya Jordan from the specific dispensing system in which each medication is stored. Locate each medication that needs to be given in this time period and click on **Put Medication on Tray** as appropriate. (*Hint:* Look in **Unit Dosage** drawer first.) When you are finished, click on **Close Drawer** and then on **View Medication Room**. Now click on the medication tray on the counter on the left side of the medication room screen to begin preparing the medications you have selected. (*Remember:* You can also click **Preparation** in the tool bar at the top of the screen.)

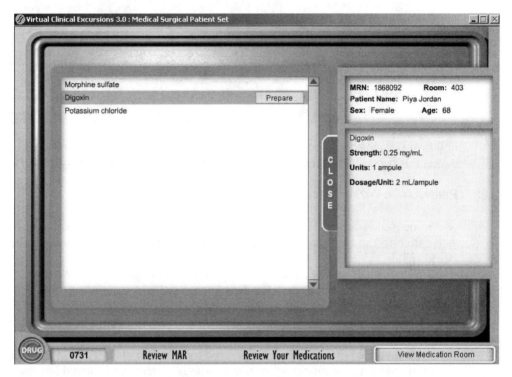

In the preparation area, you should see a list of the medications you put on the tray in the previous steps. Click on the first medication and then click **Prepare**. Follow the onscreen instructions of the Preparation Wizard, providing any data requested. As an example, let's follow the preparation process for digoxin, one of the medications due to be administered to Piya Jordan during this period of care. To begin, click to select **Digoxin**; then click **Prepare**. Now work through the Preparation Wizard sequence as detailed below:

> Amount of medication in the ampule: 2 mL.
> Enter the amount of medication you will draw up into a syringe: **0.5** mL.
> Click **Next**.
> Select the patient you wish to set aside the medication for: **Room 403, Piya Jordan**.
> Click **Finish**.
> Click **Return to Medication Room**.

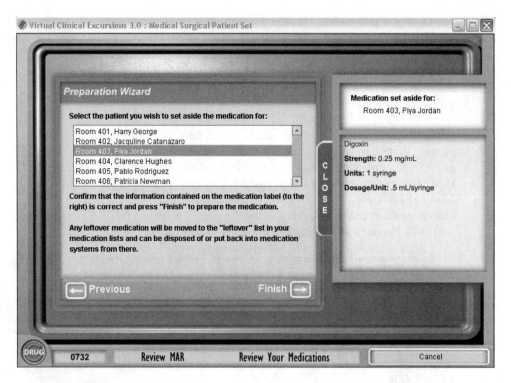

Follow this same basic process for the other medications due to be administered to Piya Jordan during this period of care. (*Hint:* Look in **IV Storage** and **Automated System**.)

PREPARATION WIZARD EXCEPTIONS

- Some medications in *Virtual Clinical Excursions* are preprepared by the pharmacy (e.g., IV antibiotics) and taken to the patient room as a whole. This is common practice in most hospitals.
- Blood products are not administered by students through the *Virtual Clinical Excursions* simulations since blood administration follows specific protocols not covered in this program.
- The *Virtual Clinical Excursions* simulations do not allow for mixing more than one type of medication, such as regular and Lente insulins, in the same syringe. In the clinical setting, when multiple types of insulin are ordered for a patient, the regular insulin is drawn up first, followed by the longer-acting insulin. Insulin is always administered in a special unit-marked syringe.

Now return to Room 403 (click on **403** on the bottom tool bar) to administer Piya Jordan's medications.

At any time during the medication administration process, you can perform a further review of systems, take vital signs, check information contained within the chart, or verify patient identity and allergies. Inside Piya Jordan's room, click **Take Vital Signs**. (*Note:* These findings change over time to reflect the temporal changes you would find in a patient similar to Piya Jordan.)

When you have gathered all the data you need, click on **Patient Care** and then select **Medication Administration**. Any medications you prepared in the previous steps should be listed on the left side of your screen. Let's continue the administration process with the digoxin ordered for Piya Jordan. Click to highlight **Digoxin** in the list of medications. Next, click on the down arrow to the right of **Select** and choose **Administer** from the drop-down menu. This will activate the Administration Wizard. Complete the Wizard sequence as follows:

- Route: **IV**
- Method: **Direct Injection**
- Site: **Peripheral IV**
- Click **Administer to Patient** arrow.
- Would you like to document this administration in the MAR? **Yes**
- Click **Finish** arrow.

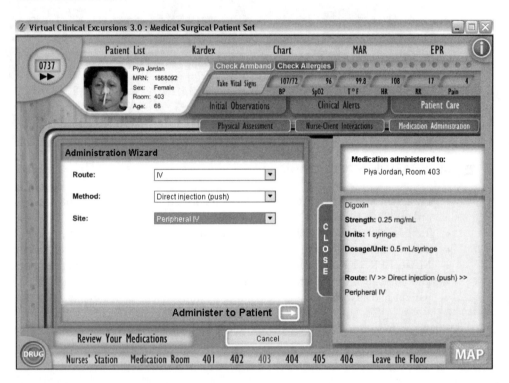

Your selections are recorded by a tracking system and evaluated on a Medication Scorecard stored under Preceptor's Evaluations. This scorecard can be viewed, printed, and given to your instructor. To access the Preceptor's Evaluations, click on **Leave the Floor**. When the Floor Menu appears, select **Look at Your Preceptor's Evaluation**. Then click on **Medication Scorecard** inside the box with Piya Jordan's name (see example on the following page).

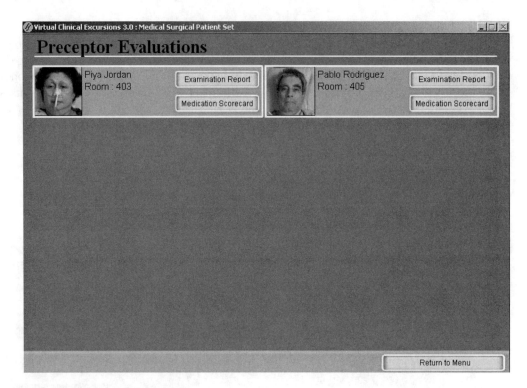

■ MEDICATION SCORECARD

- First, review Table A. Was digoxin given correctly? Did you give the other medications as ordered?
- Table B shows you which (if any) medications you gave incorrectly.
- Table C addresses the resources used for Piya Jordan. Did you access the patient's chart, MAR, EPR, or Kardex as needed to make safe medication administration decisions?
- Did you check the patient's armband to verify her identity? Did you check whether your patient had any known allergies to medications? Were vital signs taken?

When you have finished reviewing the scorecard, click **Return to Evaluations** and then **Return to Menu**.

■ **VITAL SIGNS**

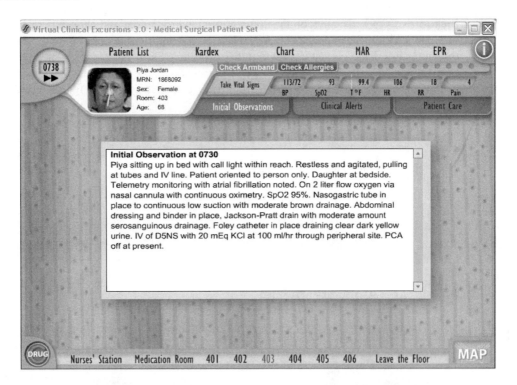

Vital signs, often considered the traditional "signs of life," include body temperature, heart rate, respiratory rate, blood pressure, oxygen saturation of the blood, and pain level.

Inside Piya Jordan's room, click **Take Vital Signs**. (*Note:* If you are following this detailed tour step by step, you will need to **Restart the Program** from the Floor Menu, sign in again, and navigate to Room 403.) Collect vital signs for this patient and record them below. Note the time at which you collected each of these data. (*Remember:* You can take vital signs at any time. The data change over time to reflect the temporal changes you would find in a patient similar to Piya Jordan.)

Vital Signs	Findings/Time
Blood pressure	
O$_2$ saturation	
Heart rate	
Respiratory rate	
Temperature	
Pain rating	

After you are done, click on the **EPR** icon located in the tool bar at the top of the screen. Your username and password are automatically provided. Click on **Login** to enter the EPR. To access Piya Jordan's records, click on the down arrow next to Patient and choose her room number, **403**. Select **Vital Signs** as the category. Next, in the empty time column on the far right, record the vital signs data you just collected in Piya Jordan's room. (*Note:* If you need help with this process, see page 16.) Now compare these findings with the data you collected earlier for this patient's vital signs. Use these earlier findings to establish a baseline for each of the vital signs.

    a.   Are any of the data you collected significantly different from the baseline for a particular vital sign?

        Circle One: Yes   No

    b.   If "Yes," which data are different?

■ PHYSICAL ASSESSMENT

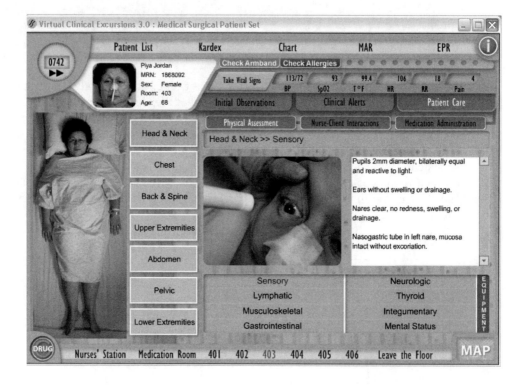

After you have finished examining the EPR for vital signs, click **Exit EPR** to return to Room 403. Click **Patient Care** and then **Physical Assessment**. Think about the information you received in the report at the beginning of this shift, as well as what you may have learned about this patient from the chart. Based on this, what area(s) of examination should you pay most attention to at this time? Is there any equipment you should be monitoring? Conduct a physical assessment of the body areas and systems that you consider priorities for Piya Jordan. For example, select **Head & Neck**; then click on and assess **Sensory** and **Lymphatic**. Complete any other assessment(s) you think are necessary at this time. In the following table, record the data you collected during this examination.

Area of Examination	Findings
Head & Neck Sensory	
Head & Neck Lymphatic	

After you have finished collecting these data, return to the EPR. Compare the data that were already in the record with those you just collected.

a. Are any of the data you collected significantly different from the baselines for this patient?

Circle One: Yes   No

b. If "Yes," which data are different?

■ NURSE-CLIENT INTERACTIONS

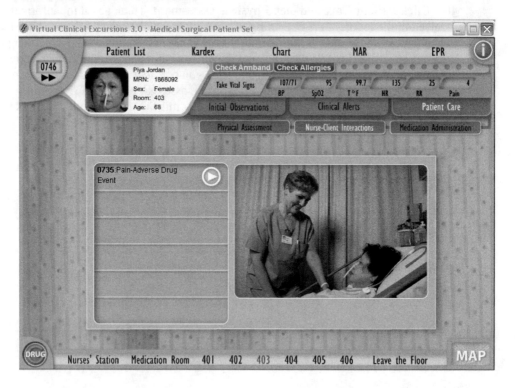

Click on **Patient Care** from inside Piya Jordan's room (403). Now click on **Nurse-Client Interactions** to access a short video titled **Pain—Adverse Drug Event**, which is available for viewing at or after 0735 (based on the virtual clock in the upper left corner of your screen; see *Note* below). To begin the video, click on the white arrow next to its title. You will observe a nurse communicating with Piya Jordan and her daughter. There are many variations of nursing practice, some exemplifying "best" practice and some not. Note whether the nurse in this interaction displays professional behavior and compassionate care. Are her words congruent with what is going on with the patient? Does this interaction "feel right" to you? If not, how would you handle this situation differently? Explain.

Note: If the video you wish to view is not listed, this means you have not yet reached the correct virtual time to view that video. Check the virtual clock; you may return to access the video once its designated time has occurred—as long as you do so within the same period of care. Or you can click on the fast-forward icon within the virtual clock to advance the time by 2-minute intervals. You will then need to click again on **Patient Care** and **Nurse-Client Interactions** to refresh the screen.

At least one Nurse-Client Interactions video is available during each period of care. Viewing these videos can help you learn more about what is occurring with a patient at a certain time and also prompt you to discern between nurse communications that are ideal and those that need improvement. Compassionate care and the ability to communicate clearly are essential components of delivering quality nursing care, and it is during your clinical time that you will begin to refine these skills.

■ COLLECTING AND EVALUATING DATA

Each of the activities you perform in the Patient Care environment generates a significant amount of assessment data. Remember that after you collect data, you can record your findings in the EPR. You can also review the EPR, patient's chart, videos, and MAR at any time. You will get plenty of practice collecting and then evaluating data in context of the patient's course.

Now, here's an important question for you:

> Did the previous sequence of exercises provide the most efficient way to assess Piya Jordan?

For example, you went to the patient's room to get vital signs, then back to the EPR to enter data and compare your findings with extant data. Next, you went back to the patient's room to do a physical examination, then again back to the EPR to enter and review data. If this back-and-forth process of data collection and recording seemed inefficient, remember the following:

- Plan all of your nursing activities to maximize efficiency, while at the same time optimizing the quality of patient care. (Think about what data you might need before performing certain tasks. For example, do you need to check a heart rate before administering a cardiac medication or check an IV site before starting an infusion?)

- You collect a tremendous amount of data when you work with a patient. Very few people can accurately remember all these data for more than a few minutes. Develop efficient assessment skills, and record data as soon as possible after collecting them.

- Assessment data are only the starting point for the nursing process.

Make a clear distinction between these first exercises and how you actually provide nursing care. These initial exercises were designed to involve you actively in the use of different software components. This workbook focuses on sensible practices for implementing the nursing process in ways that ensure the highest-quality care of patients.

Most important, remember that a human being changes through time, and that these changes include both the physical and psychosocial facets of a person as a living organism. Think about this for a moment. Some patients may change physically in a very short time (a patient with emerging myocardial infarction) or more slowly (a patient with a chronic illness). Patients' overall physical and psychosocial conditions may improve or deteriorate. They may have effective coping skills and familial support, or they may feel alone and full of despair. In fact, each individual is a complex mix of physical and psychosocial elements, and at least some of these elements usually change through time.

Thus it is crucial that you *DO NOT* think of the nursing process as a simple one-time, five-step procedure consisting of assessment, nursing diagnosis, planning, implementation, and evaluation. Rather, the nursing process should be utilized as a creative and systematic approach to delivering nursing care. Furthermore, because all living organisms are constantly changing, we must apply the nursing process over and over. Each time we follow the nursing process for an individual patient, we refine our understanding of that patient's physical and psychosocial conditions based on collection and analysis of many different types of data. *Virtual Clinical Excursions* will help you develop both the creativity and the systematic approach needed to become a nurse who is equipped to deliver the highest-quality care to all patients.

REDUCING MEDICATION ERRORS

Earlier in this detailed tour, you learned the basic steps of medication preparation and administration. The following simulations will allow you to practice those skills further—with an increased emphasis on reducing medication errors by using the Medication Scorecard to evaluate your work.

Using the *Virtual Clinical Excursions—Medical-Surgical* program (Disk 2), sign in to work at Pacific View Regional Hospital for Period of Care 1. (*Note:* If you are already working with another patient or during another period of care, click on **Leave the Floor** and then **Restart the Program**; then sign in.)

From the Patient List, select Clarence Hughes. Then click on **Go to Nurses' Station**. Complete the following steps to prepare and administer medications to Clarence Hughes.

- Click on **Medication Room**.
- Click on **MAR** and then on tab **404** to determine prn medications that have been ordered for Clarence Hughes. (*Note:* You may click on **Review MAR** at any time to verify the correct medication order. Always remember to check the patient name on the MAR to make sure you have the correct patient's record—you must click on the correct room number tab within the MAR.) Click on **Return to Medication Room** after reviewing the correct MAR.
- Click on **Unit Dosage** (or on the Unit Dosage cabinet); from the close-up view, click on drawer **404**.
- Select the medications you would like to administer. After each selection, click **Put Medication on Tray**. When you are finished selecting medications, click **Close Drawer** and then **View Medication Room**.
- Click on **Automated System** (or on the Automated System unit itself). Click **Login**.
- On the next screen, specify the correct patient and drawer location.
- Select the medication you would like to administer and click on **Put Medication on Tray**. Repeat this process if you wish to administer other medications from the Automated System.
- When you are finished, click **Close Drawer** and **View Medication Room**.
- From the Medication Room, click on **Preparation** (or on the preparation tray).
- From the list of medications on your tray, highlight the correct medication to administer and click **Prepare**.
- This activates the Preparation Wizard. Supply any requested information; then click **Next**.
- Now select the correct patient to receive this medication and click **Finish**.
- Repeat the previous three steps until all medications that you want to administer are prepared.
- You can click on **Review Your Medications** and then on **Return to Medication Room** when ready. Once you are back in the Medication Room, go directly to Clarence Hughes' room by clicking on **404** at bottom of screen.
- Inside the patient's room, administer the medication, utilizing the five rights of medication administration. After you have collected the appropriate assessment data and are ready for administration, click **Patient Care** and then **Medication Administration**. Verify that the correct patient and medication(s) appear in the left-hand window. Highlight the first medication you wish to administer; then click the down arrow next to Select. From the drop-down menu, select **Administer** and complete the Administration Wizard by providing any information requested. When the Wizard stops asking for information, click **Administer to Patient**. Specify **Yes** when asked whether this administration should be recorded in the MAR. Finally, click **Finish**.

■ **SELF-EVALUATION**

Now let's see how you did during your medication administration!

- Click on **Leave the Floor** at the bottom of your screen. From the Floor Menu, select **Look at Your Preceptor's Evaluation**. Then click **Medication Scorecard**.

The following exercises will help you identify medication errors, investigate possible reasons for these errors, and reduce or prevent medication errors in the future.

1. Start by examining Table A. These are the medications you should have given to Clarence Hughes during this period of care. If each of the medications in Table A has a ✓ by it, then you made no errors. Congratulations!

If any medication has an X by it, then you made one or more medication errors.

Compare Tables A and B to determine which of the following types of errors you made: Wrong Dose, Wrong Route/Method/Site, or Wrong Time. Follow these steps:
   a. Find medications in Table A that were given incorrectly.
   b. Now see if those same medications are in Table B, which shows what you actually administered to Clarence Hughes.
   c. Comparing Tables A and B, match the Strength, Dose, Route/Method/Site, and Time for each medication you administered incorrectly.
   d. Then, using the form below, list the medications given incorrectly and mark the errors you made for each medication.

Medication	Strength	Dosage	Route	Method	Site	Time
	❑	❑	❑	❑	❑	❑
	❑	❑	❑	❑	❑	❑
	❑	❑	❑	❑	❑	❑
	❑	❑	❑	❑	❑	❑

2. To help you reduce future medication errors, consider the following list of possible reasons for errors.

- Did not check drug against MAR for correct patient, correct date, correct time, correct drug, and correct dose.
- Did not check drug dose against MAR three times.
- Did not open the unit dose package in the patient's room.
- Did not correctly identify the patient using two identifiers.
- Did not administer the drug on time.
- Did not verify patient allergies.
- Did not check the patient's current condition or vital sign parameters.
- Did not consider why the patient would be receiving this drug.
- Did not question why the drug was in the patient's drawer.
- Did not check the physician's order and/or check with the pharmacist when there was a question about the drug or dose.
- Did not verify that no adverse effects had occurred from a previous dose.

Based on the list of possibilities you just reviewed, determine how you made each error and record the reason in the form below:

Medication	Reason for Error

3. Look again at Table B. Are there medications listed that are not in Table A? If so, you gave a medication to Clarence Hughes that he should not have received. Complete the following exercises to help you understand how such an error might have been made.

    a. Perhaps you gave a medication that was on Clarence Hughes' MAR for this period of care, without recognizing that a change had occurred in the patient's condition, which should have caused you to reconsider. Review patient records as necessary and complete the following form:

Medication	Possible Reasons Not to Give This Medication

    b. Another possibility is that you gave Clarence Hughes a medication that should have been given at a different time. Check his MAR and complete the form below to determine whether you made a Wrong Time error:

Medication	Given to Clarence Hughes at What Time	Should Have Been Given at What Time

c. Maybe you gave another patient's medication to Clarence Hughes. In this case, you made a Wrong Patient error. Check the MARs of other patients and use the form below to determine whether you made this type of error:

Medication	Given to Clarence Hughes	Should Have Been Given to

4. The Medication Scorecard provides some other interesting sources of information. For example, if there is a medication selected for Clarence Hughes but it was not given to him, there will be an X by that medication in Table A, but it will not appear in Table B. In that case, you might have given this medication to some other patient, which is another type of Wrong Patient error. To investigate further, look at Table D, which lists the medications you gave to other patients. See whether you can find any medications ordered for Clarence Hughes that were given to another patient by mistake. However, before you make any decisions, be sure to cross-check the MAR for other patients because the same medication may have been ordered for multiple patients. Use the following form to record your findings:

Medication	Should Have Been Given to Clarence Hughes	Given by Mistake to

5. Now take some time to review the medication exercises you just completed. Use the form below to create an overall analysis of what you have learned. Once again, record each of the medication errors you made, including the type of each error. Then, for each error you made, indicate specifically what you would do differently to prevent this type of error from occurring again.

Medication	Type of Error	Error Prevention Tactic

Submit this form to your instructor if required as a graded assignment, or simply use these exercises to improve your understanding of medication errors and how to reduce them.

Name: _____ Date: _____

The following icons are used throughout this workbook to help you quickly identify particular activities and assignments:

 Indicates a reading assignment—tells you which textbook chapter(s) you should read before starting each lesson

 Indicates a writing activity

 Marks the beginning of an interactive CD-ROM activity—signals you to open or return to your *Virtual Clinical Excursions* CD-ROM

 Indicates additional CD-ROM instructions

 Indicates questions and activities that require you to consult your textbook

 Indicates the approximate time required to complete an exercise

LESSON **1**

An Overview of Communication Barriers

Reading Assignment: Communication (Chapter 3)

Patient: William Jefferson, Room 501 (Disk 1)

Objectives:

1. Identify the factors that may hinder nurse-patient interactions.
2. List the communication tools necessary to successfully interact with cognitively impaired patients.
3. Discuss three styles of communication.
4. Understand the rationale for nursing interventions used to successfully communicate with cognitively impaired patients.

Exercise 1

 Writing Activity

 30 minutes

   1. List some obstacles that may affect interactions between nurses and older adult patients.

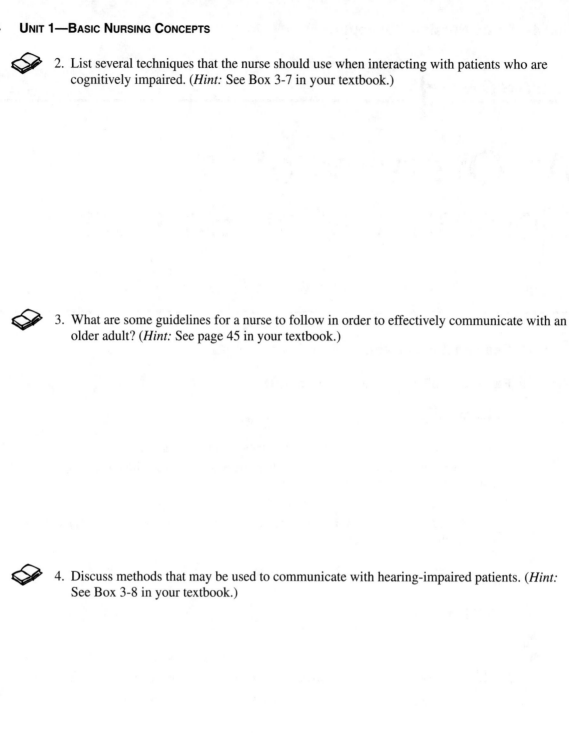

2. List several techniques that the nurse should use when interacting with patients who are cognitively impaired. (*Hint:* See Box 3-7 in your textbook.)

3. What are some guidelines for a nurse to follow in order to effectively communicate with an older adult? (*Hint:* See page 45 in your textbook.)

4. Discuss methods that may be used to communicate with hearing-impaired patients. (*Hint:* See Box 3-8 in your textbook.)

5. The two types of communication are _____ and _____.

6. List the elements of nonverbal communication. (*Hint:* See Box 3-1 in your textbook.)

7. A therapeutic nurse-patient interaction is necessary to promote quality care. Which of the following elements foster a therapeutic client to nurse relationship? Select all that apply.

_____ Hugging

_____ Sincerity

_____ Empathy

_____ Trustworthiness

_____ Sympathy

_____ Demonstrating parental behaviors toward the patient

_____ Caring attitude

8. _____ refers to a communication technique that incorporates the feelings and needs of the patient.

9. The communication style that overpowers the other member(s) in the interaction is

_____ communication.

10. Which of the following behaviors by the nurse demonstrate cultural awareness when caring for a patient? Select all that apply.

_____ Maintain eye contact during the interaction.

_____ Use touch as appropriate for the interaction after patient comfort level has been assessed.

_____ Call the patient by his or her first name to promote feelings of familiarity and closeness.

_____ Assess contextual speech patterns of the patient's cultural group.

_____ Identify personal spatial and distancing characteristics employed by the patient.

11. What must the nurse take into consideration when using touch to communicate with a patient? (*Hint:* See page 38 in your textbook.)

12. What should a nurse understand regarding a patient's beliefs and/or decisions?

13. Which of the following guidelines must be remembered when using humor during a patient interaction?
    a. There must be a mutual comfort level between the patient and nurse.
    b. Humor should not be used during periods of emotional grief.
    c. The nurse should be the party leading the interaction and determining when the use of humor is appropriate.
    d. Humor cannot be used during periods in which the patient is experiencing pain.

Exercise 2

 CD-ROM Activity

 15 minutes

- Using the *Virtual Clinical Excursions—Skilled Nursing* CD (Disk 1), sign in to work at Pacific View Regional Hospital for Period of Care 1. (*Note:* If you are already in the virtual hospital from a previous exercise, click on **Leave the Floor** and then **Restart the Program** to get to the sign-in window.)
- From the Patient List, select William Jefferson (Room 501).
- Click on **Get Report** and read the Clinical Report.
- Click on **Go to Nurses' Station**; then click on **501** to go to the patient's room.
- Review the Initial Observation notes.

1. What psychosocial issues could affect the nurse's interaction with William Jefferson? How might these behaviors affect the interaction?

2. What physiologic and environmental issues being experienced by William Jefferson may affect the nurse-patient interaction?

3. Which of the following interventions will assist the nurse in establishing a positive rapport when communicating with William Jefferson? Select all that apply.

   _____ Assist the patient to the dining room to promote feelings of socialization.

   _____ Face him during the interaction.

   _____ Avoid analgesic administration to reduce drowsiness during the interaction.

   _____ Provide adequate lighting during the exchange.

   _____ Use touch as culturally appropriate.

4. When the nurse is caring for William Jefferson, which of the following variables will have the most influence on communication?
   a. His age and race
   b. His culture and social position
   c. Scheduled agenda for the day
   d. Race of the care provider
   e. Disorientation and confusion

Exercise 3

 CD-ROM Activity

 15 minutes

- Using the *Virtual Clinical Excursions—Skilled Nursing* CD (Disk 1), sign in to work at Pacific View Regional Hospital for Period of Care 2. (*Note:* If you are already in the virtual hospital from a previous exercise, click on **Leave the Floor** and then **Restart the Program** to get to the sign-in window.)
- From the Patient List, select William Jefferson (Room 501).
- Click on **Get Report** and read the Clinical Report.

1. What cognitive changes have taken place in William Jefferson during the last shift?

2. What behavioral manifestations are occurring as a result of these changes?

 • Click on **Go to Nurses' Station** and then on **501**.
- Review the Initial Observation notes.
- Click on **Patient Care** and then on **Nurse-Client Interactions**.
- Select and view the video titled **1115: Team Communication**. (*Note:* Check the virtual clock to see whether enough time has elapsed. You can use the fast-forward feature to advance the time by 2-minute intervals if the video is not yet available. Then click on **Patient Care** and **Nurse-Client Interactions** to refresh the screen.)

3. What three planned nursing interventions were discussed in the team conference that will be implemented by the nurse?

4. Give a rationale for each of the planned interventions in question 3.

 •   Now select and view the video titled **1120: The Agitated Patient**. (*Note:* Check the virtual clock to see whether enough time has elapsed. You can use the fast-forward feature to advance the time by 2-minute intervals if the video is not yet available. Then click on **Patient Care** and **Nurse-Client Interactions** to refresh the screen.)

5. In the video, what verbal communication technique does the nurse use in her interaction with William Jefferson?

6. What were the nonverbal cues used during the nurse's interaction with the patient?

 7. Which of the following factors associated with the patient's room may affect communication? (*Hint:* See pages 43-44 in your textbook.)
    a. The color of the room (may trigger negative feelings)
    b. The size of the room
    c. The physical layout of the room
    d. The lack of a roommate

8. What did the nurse do to reinforce William Jefferson's mental orientation?

LESSON 2 ‗‗‗‗‗‗‗‗‗‗‗‗‗‗‗‗‗‗‗‗‗‗‗‗‗‗‗‗‗‗

The Nursing Assessment

‗‗‗‗‗‗‗‗‗‗‗‗‗‗‗‗‗‗‗‗‗‗‗‗‗‗‗‗‗‗‗‗‗‗‗‗‗‗

Reading Assignment: Physical Assessment (Chapter 4)

Patient: William Jefferson, Room 501 (Disk 1)

Objectives:

1. Discuss the role of the shift report and explain its importance.
2. Discuss the assessment techniques that may be used when performing a physical assessment.
3. Review the two techniques that may be used to perform a comprehensive nursing assessment.
4. Identify abnormal findings on a physical examination.

Exercise 1

 Writing Activity

 15 minutes

 1. What is the purpose of the shift report (also called the change-of-shift report)? (*Hint:* See pages 2115-2116 in your textbook.)

2. Which of the following elements is *most* necessary when performing a shift report?
   a. Accuracy of information
   b. Information concerning the patient's personality
   c. Information regarding the patient's family support
   d. The nurse's opinion about the patient's family background

51

3. What elements should not be included in the shift report?

4. The shift report should include which of the following elements to promote positive communication between members of the health care team? Select all that apply.

_____ Accurate information

_____ Information concerning the patient's personality

_____ Information regarding the level of the patient's family support

_____ The nurse's personal feelings about the patient

_____ The nurse's opinions about the patient's family background

5. What is the purpose of the nursing assessment?

6. What environmental considerations should be included in the physical assessment?

7. If you are approaching a patient for the first time to perform an assessment, what preliminary steps must you take.

8. What are the two techniques used to perform a comprehensive nursing assessment?

 9. Match each assessment technique with its definitions. (*Hint:* See Box 4-4 in your textbook.)

Assessment Technique	Definition
_____ Inspection	a. The use of the fingertips to tap the body's surface and produce vibration and sound
_____ Palpation	b. A visual observation of the patient's body, responses to questioning, and nonverbal behaviors
_____ Ascultation	c. The use of the hands and sense of touch to gather information
_____ Percussion	d. The process of listening to sounds produced by the body

Exercise 2

 CD-ROM Activity

 45 minutes

- Using the *Virtual Clinical Excursions—Skilled Nursing* CD (Disk 1), sign in to work at Pacific View Regional Hospital for Period of Care 2. (*Note:* If you are already in the virtual hospital from a previous exercise, click on **Leave the Floor** and then **Restart the Program** to get to the sign-in window.)
- From the Patient List, select William Jefferson (Room 501).
- Click on **Get Report** and read the Clinical Report.
- Click on **Go to Nurses' Station**.
- Click on **501** to go to the patient's room; then click on **Patient Care**.

1. Which manner of data collection is being used by the nurse to assess William Jefferson?

→ • Click on **Head & Neck** and review the assessment data in each area.

2. What tools are needed to complete this assessment? (*Hint:* See page 69 in your textbook.)

3. List any abnormal findings in the nurse's assessment of William Jefferson's head and neck.

4. What clues can be obtained from the examination of the mouth and teeth? (*Hint:* See page 69 in your textbook.)

5. When the pupils are equal and reactive to light, what acronym is used?

→ • Click on **Chest** and review the assessment data in each area.

6. List any abnormal findings in the nurse's assessment of William Jefferson's chest.

7. Match each adventitious lung sound with its description.

Lung Sound	Description of Sound
_____ Crackles	a. Sounds produced by a narrowing in the airway passages
_____ Wheezes	b. Bubbling sounds that may be evidenced on inspiration
_____ Pleural friction rubs	c. Sounds produced by inflammation in the pleural sac—may have a rubbing, grating, or friction sound

8. Heart sounds should be assessed for _____ and _____. (*Hint:* See page 72 in your textbook.)

→ • Click on **Back & Spine** and review the assessment data in each area.

9. List any abnormal findings in the nurse's assessment of William Jefferson's back and spine.

→ • Click on **Upper Extremities** and review the assessment data in each area.

10. Identify any unusual findings in the assessment of the upper extremities.

11. During an assessment of the abdomen, the patient's knees should be

_____.

12. Which of the following is the optimal positioning of a patient during an abdominal assessment? (*Hint:* See page 73 in your textbook.)
   a. Supine
   b. Prone
   c. Trendelenburg

13. Match the following columns to show the appropriate sequence of events for assessing a patient's abdomen.

Action	**Order in Sequence**
_____ Auscultate for bowel sounds in each of the four quadrants	a. First
	b. Second
_____ Palpate for masses or other abnormalities	c. Third
_____ Visually inspect the abdomen for size, symmetry, and general appearance	

➤ • Click on **Lower Extremities** and review the assessment data in each area.

14. List any findings of interest in the assessment of William Jefferson's lower extremities.

15. How is the capillary refill test performed?

16. William Jefferson's capillary refill is noted to be sluggish. What are potential causes of this finding?

3

The Nursing Process

 Reading Assignment: Nursing Process and Critical Thinking (Chapter 5)

Patient: William Jefferson, Room 501 (Disk 1)

Objectives:

1. Identify sources of data when developing a plan of care.
2. Discuss the differences between nursing and medical diagnoses.
3. Apply the principles of the nursing process.
4. Prioritize the patient concerns by level of importance.

Exercise 1

 Writing Activity

15 minutes

   1. Explain the differences between subjective and objective data.

2. In addition to the patient, who and/or what are some other sources of data?

3. What is the purpose of a nursing diagnosis, and what are the four components of a nursing diagnosis? (*Hint:* See pages 84-86 in your textbook.)

4. How do medical and nursing diagnoses differ?

5. Match each aspect of the nursing process with its appropriate description.

Nursing Process Aspect	Description
_____ Assess	a. Set goals of care and desired outcomes
_____ Plan and identify outcomes	b. Identify the patient's problems
_____ Implement	c. Gather information about the patient's condition
_____ Evaluate	d. Determine whether goals are met and outcomes have been achieved
_____ Diagnose	e. Perform the nursing actions identified in planning

Exercise 2

 CD-ROM Activity

 45 minutes

- Using the *Virtual Clinical Excursions—Skilled Nursing* CD (Disk 1), sign in to work at Pacific View Regional Hospital for Period of Care 3. (*Note:* If you are already in the virtual program from a previous exercise, click on **Leave the Floor** and then **Restart the Program** to get to the sign-in window.)
- From the Patient List, select William Jefferson (Room 501).
- Click on **Get Report** and read the Clinical Report.
- Click on **Go to Nurses' Station** and then on **Chart**.
- Click on **501** to open William Jefferson's chart.
- Click on the **Nursing Admission** tab and read the report.

1. Who appears to be the primary provider of information in the nursing admission assessment of William Jefferson?

2. Identify the primary concerns reported by the patient.

3. Which of the following have been identified as medical diagnoses for William Jefferson? Select all that apply.

_____ Alzheimer's disease

_____ Stress incontinence

_____ Urinary tract infection

_____ Hypertension

_____ Potential for anxiety

_____ Osteoarthritis

_____ Type 2 diabetes

_____ Diabetes insipidus

_____ Resolving sepsis

→ • Click on the **History and Physical** tab and review the report.

4. Based on information collected in the Nursing Admission and the History and Physical, identify several areas of concern for William Jefferson.

5. For three of the above areas of concern, develop possible nursing diagnoses.

6. _____ statements are based on the desired patient-driven expectations.

7. Patient-driven outcomes are referred to as _____.

8. The system used to prioritize the needs of a patient, with physiologic needs coming before

   those focusing on love and belonging, is known as _____.

9. Listed below are the identified areas of concern for William Jefferson. Rank them in order of importance.

Area of Concern	Order of Importance
_____ Potential for reinfection	a. First
_____ Management and stabilization of hypertension	b. Second
	c. Third
_____ Management and stabilization of diabetes mellitus	

10. Develop a patient outcome relating to William Jefferson's potential for injury.

11. Develop a patient outcome relating to William Jefferson's diabetes mellitus.

12. How do nursing interventions and physician-prescribed interventions differ?

→ • Click on the **Physician's Orders** tab and review the orders for Tuesday at 1230.

13. Which of the orders listed below are nursing interventions? Select all that apply.

_____ Temperature, pulse, respirations daily only

_____ Fingerstick capillary glucose at bedtime tonight

_____ Fasting blood glucose Wednesday morning

_____ Continue blood pressure check every 8 hours

→ • Click on the **Consultations** tab and review the data.

14. Why are multiple disciplines utilized to provide care to a patient?

15. What consultations have been made so far in William Jefferson's care?

16. Based on the data presented, what additional consultations might be helpful to William Jefferson and his family?

17. Based on the data presented concerning William Jefferson's physical condition and psychosocial needs, which of the following consultations would be helpful to him and his family? Select all that apply.

_____ Support groups

_____ Respite care resources

_____ Respiratory therapy

_____ Cardiovascular rehabilitation

_____ Dietary consultation

LESSON 4 _____

Establishment of End-of-Life Wishes

_____

👓 **Reading Assignment:** Loss, Grief, Dying, and Death (Chapter 9)

Patient: Goro Oishi, Room 505 (Disk 1)

Objectives:

1. Discuss the concepts of an advance directive.
2. Develop nursing diagnoses for the family of the dying patient.
3. Discuss the emotional support needed by the family members of a dying patient.
4. List potential referrals for the family experiencing an impending death.

Exercise 1

 Writing Activity

 15 minutes

1. A legal document that outlines the health care wishes of a patient in the event that the patient becomes unable to make decisions is referred to as:
   a. an advance directive.
   b. a power of attorney.
   c. a guardianship.
   d. a health care liaison.

2. What is required to make the above document legal and binding? Select all that apply.

_____ The document must be signed and dated by the patient.

_____ The signing must be witnessed by two health care providers.

_____ The document must be reviewed and approved by the physician.

_____ The signing must be witnessed by two people who will not inherit any property upon the patient's death.

_____ The signing must be witnessed by two family members of the patient.

_____ The patient must seek spiritual counseling before signing the document.

3. How does a Do Not Resuscitate (DNR) order affect the nurse's care?

4. A document that directs medical treatment in accordance with a patient's wishes in the event of a terminal illness or condition is called a _____.

5. The designation of a person other than the patient to make health care decisions on the patient's behalf is called a _____.

Exercise 2

 CD-ROM Activity

 45 minutes

- Using the *Virtual Clinical Excursions—Skilled Nursing* CD (Disk 1), sign in to work at Pacific View Regional Hospital for Period of Care 1. (*Note:* If you are already in the virtual hospital from a previous exercise, click on **Leave the Floor** and then **Restart the Program** to get to the sign-in window.)
- From the Patient List, select Goro Oishi (Room 505).
- Click on **Get Report** and read the Clinical Report.
- Click on **Go to Nurses' Station** and then on **Chart**.
- Click on **505** to view Goro Oishi's chart.
- Click on the **History and Physical** tab and review the report.

1. Why was Goro Oishi admitted to the hospital, and what is his current status?

2. What elements have been identified in his plan of care?

 - Click on the **Physician's Notes** tab and read the progress notes.
- Next, click on the **Consents** tab and review the information given.

3. Who is in control of Goro Oishi's medical care, and why is this person able to direct his care?

4. Which of the following statements regarding the roles of those in charge of Goro Oishi's health care is correct?
   a. Mrs. Oishi will have the authority to handle her husband's financial affairs.
   b. Mrs. Oishi will be required to consult with the entire family to obtain a consensus when making critical decisions.
   c. The physician will be required to make the final determination regarding the health care decisions.
   d. The Oishi family attorney will be required to go to court to make Mrs. Oishi her husband's health care guardian.
   e. Mrs. Oishi can make all of the health care decisions in the event that her husband is unable to make decisions for himself.

5. What provisions have been made in the event that Mrs. Oishi is unable to accept the role?

6. _____ If Goro Oishi's son does not agree with Mrs. Oishi, her wishes may be considered invalid. (True or False)

7. List the specific powers given to Mrs. Oishi by the advance directive.

8. Ideally, who should be given copies of an advance directive prior to its being implemented? Select all that apply.

   _____ Members of the immediate family

   _____ A judge

   _____ The primary physician

   _____ The family's attorney

   _____ The nurses providing care

9. List the health care decisions that were addressed by Goro Oishi's advance directive.

→ • Click on the **Consultations** tab and review the information given.

10. What referrals have been made to assist the Oishi family at this time?

11. What was the outcome of this consultation?

→ • Click on the **Nurse's Notes** tab and review the notes.

12. Discuss the family's support of Goro Oishi's health care directives.

13. Identify one goal and outcome for the Oishi family during the dying process.

14. Develop a nursing diagnosis for the Oishi family during the dying process.

LESSON *5*

Care of the Dying Patient

⌒⌒ **Reading Assignment:** Loss, Grief, Dying, and Death (Chapter 9)

Patient: Goro Oishi, Room 505 (Disk 1)

Objectives:

1. Define palliative care.
2. List the priority needs of the dying patient.
3. Recognize the physiologic signs and symptoms of impending death.
4. List the clinical signs of death.
5. Identify nursing interventions in the care of the dying patient.

Exercise 1

Writing Activity

 15 minutes

1. Identify the three most important needs of the dying patient.

2. _____ is the provision of care to promote comfort of a
   dying patient. Measures are not geared toward sustaining life.

3. List the changes that occur in vital signs of the patient with impending death.

 4. Describe the progression of neurologic and motor changes in a patient as death becomes closer. (*Hint:* See page 209 in your textbook.)

5. _____ As death draws closer, there is typically diminished sensory and motor function in the lower extremities that progresses to the upper extremities. (True or False)

6. List the clinical signs of death.

7. Which of the following is characteristic of the concept of death for most adults between the ages of 45 and 65 years? (*Hint:* See Table 9-2 in your textbook.)
   a. Fears of a long and lingering death
   b. Attitudes that are influenced by cultural beliefs
   c. Belief that death will allow freedom from pain and a reunion with deceased family and friends
   d. Acceptance of one's own mortality

Exercise 2

 CD-ROM Activity

 30 minutes

- Using the *Virtual Clinical Excursions—Skilled Nursing* CD (Disk 1), sign in to work at Pacific View Regional Hospital for Period of Care 1. (*Note:* If you are already in the virtual hospital from a previous exercise, click on **Leave the Floor** and then **Restart the Program** to get to the sign-in window.)
- From the Patient List, select Goro Oishi (Room 505).
- Click on **Get Report** and read the Clinical Report.
- Click on **Go to Nurses' Station** and then on **505** to enter the patient's room.
- Click on **Initial Observations** and review.
- Next, click on **Take Vital Signs**.

  1. List Goro Oishi's vital signs.

     BP:

     Temp:

     HR:

     RR:

     SpO$_2$:

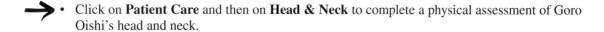 - Click on **Patient Care** and then on **Head & Neck** to complete a physical assessment of Goro Oishi's head and neck.

  2. Which findings in the head and neck assessment are consistent with Goro Oishi's comatose and brain-damaged status?

 - Click on **Chest** and complete a physical assessment.

  3. What finding in the chest assessment supports the comatose diagnosis?

→ • Click on the remaining sections of the head-to-toe assessment and review the notes for each.

4. What additional findings in the remainder of the assessment support the diagnosis?

5. Discuss Goro Oishi's urinary output.

→ • Click on **Chart** and then on **505** to view Goro Oishi's chart.
 • Click on the **Physician's Orders** tab to review the orders.

6. Several interventions have been ordered to promote Goro Oishi's level of comfort. For each rationale listed below, enter the intervention ordered.

a. To assist with respiratory function and promote comfort, _____

_____.

b. To aid in maintaining oxygenation and reduce respiratory distress, _____

_____ has been ordered.

c. To reduce respiratory distress and choking potential, _____.

d. To decrease discomfort associated with drying of the mucous membranes, _____

_____.

e. To reduce fever and promote comfort, administer _____.

f. To increase Goro Oishi's level of comfort, perform _____ TID.

7. As noted, Goro Oishi has a "DNR" order in place. What is the purpose of the other orders concerning his care?

Exercise 3

 CD-ROM Activity

 15 minutes

- Using the *Virtual Clinical Excursions—Skilled Nursing* CD (Disk 1), sign in to work at Pacific View Regional Hospital for Period of Care 3. (*Note:* If you are already in the virtual hospital from the previous exercise, click on **Leave the Floor** and then **Restart the Program** to get to the sign-in window.)
- From the Patient List, select Goro Oishi (Room 505).
- Click on **Get Report** and read the Clinical Report.
- Click on **Go to Nurses' Station** and then on **505** to enter the patient's room.
- Review the Initial Observation notes.

1. What physiologic changes have take place during the previous shift?

 - Click on **Take Vital Signs** and review.

2. Describe the changes noted in the patient's vital signs and discuss the implications of each.

→ • Click on **Patient Care** and then on **Head & Neck** to complete a physical assessment of Goro Oishi's head and neck.

3. What significant changes have taken place that are manifested in the assessment of the head and neck?

4. What findings indicate a reduction in cardiopulmonary functioning?

5. Develop a nursing diagnosis for the Oishi family during this period.

6. What care interventions to the family are appropriate at this time?

LESSON **6**

Assessment of Vital Signs

 Reading Assignment: Vital Signs (Chapter 11)

Patient: Kathryn Doyle, Room 503 (Disk 1)

Objectives:

1. Recognize abnormal vital sign readings.
2. List the factors that will affect vital sign readings.
3. Discuss the actions that should be taken when abnormal readings are observed.
4. Discuss the use of pharmacologic agents in the management of febrile states.

Exercise 1

 Writing Activity

15 minutes

  1. List several factors that could cause an elevation in temperature.

  2. The _____ regulates body temperature by maintaining a balance between heat lost and heat produced by the body.

3. How does the time of day affect the body's temperature reading?

4. When referring to a patient with an elevated temperature, which of the following terms may be used? Select all that apply.

_____ Afebrile

_____ Hyposphresia

_____ Febrile

_____ Hyperthermic

_____ Pyretic

5. List several signs and symptoms that may accompany an elevated temperature. (*Hint:* See Box 11-5 in your textbook.)

6. _____ The metabolic rate will increase if the body's temperature is elevated. (True or False)

7. Which of the following are not indications for using an electronic blood pressure monitoring tool? Check all that apply.

_____ Irregular heart rate

_____ Excessive patient fatigue

_____ Patients having a slender build

_____ Seizure activity

_____ Peripheral vascular obstructions

8. In addition to an elevated temperature, what other factors may affect the pulse rate? (*Hint:* See Box 11-8 in your textbook.)

9. _____ is the term used to indicate an elevation in the pulse rate.

Exercise 2

 CD-ROM Activity

 45 minutes

- Using the *Virtual Clinical Excursions—Skilled Nursing* CD (Disk 1), sign in to work at Pacific View Regional Hospital for Period of Care 1. (*Note:* If you are already in the virtual hospital from a previous exercise, click on **Leave the Floor** and **Restart the Program** to get to the sign-in window.)
- From the Patient List, select Kathryn Doyle (Room 503).
- Click on **Get Report** and read the Clinical Report.
- Click on **Go to Nurses' Station** then on **503** to enter the patient's room.
- Click on **Take Vital Signs**.

1. What are Kathryn Doyle's vital signs?

    Temp:

    BP:

    HR:

    RR:

2. Discuss any abnormal findings in the above vital signs.

3. Based on your knowledge of Kathryn Doyle's health history, to what might her elevated temperature be attributed?

4. What interventions may be utilized to treat Kathryn Doyle's temperature elevation?

5. _____ Since Kathryn Doyle's temperature is elevated, her heart rate will be decreased. (True or False)

6. If a nursing assistant is available to assist in taking Kathryn Doyle's vital signs, which of the following statements is **most** correct?
   a. The nursing assistant may be delegated the responsibility of taking the vital signs.
   b. Since there is an abnormality in Kathryn Doyle's vital signs, the nursing assistant should not be delegated this particular patient.
   c. The nursing assistant may take the vital signs, but charting the findings is the responsibility of the nurse.
   d. Although the nursing assistant may be delegated the responsibility of taking the vital signs, the nurse is still responsible for monitoring the results.

 • Click on **Patient Care** and then on **Nurse-Client Interactions**.
   • Select and view the video titled **0730: Assessment—Biopsychosocial**. (*Note:* Check the virtual clock to see whether enough time has elapsed. You can use the fast-forward feature to advance the time by 2-minute intervals if the video is not yet available. Then click on **Patient Care** and **Nurse-Client Interactions** to refresh the screen.)

7. In the video, what actions and/or statements by Kathryn Doyle support the elevated temperature finding?

8. Discuss the impact that Kathryn Doyle's elevated temperature will have on the frequency of her assessments.

9. Which of the following actions should the nurse take prior to reporting the elevation in Kathryn Doyle's temperature?

_____ Recheck the temperature to ensure proper functioning of equipment.

_____ Administer acetaminophen.

_____ Check physician's orders to determine whether call orders have been left.

_____ Ask a nursing assistant to recheck the temperature.

_____ Ask the patient whether she had eaten just before her temperature was taken.

_____ Give the patient a tepid sponge bath.

_____ Administer ordered antibiotics.

→ • Click on **Chart** and then on **503** to view Kathryn Doyle's chart.
   • Click on the **Physician's Orders** tab and review the orders.

10. What orders has the physician left regarding Kathryn Doyle's temperature?

11. Prior to administration of acetaminophen, what actions should the nurse take?

12. Which of Kathryn Doyle's prescribed medications may have had an impact on her current temperature?

_____ Ferrous sulfate

_____ Calcium citrate

_____ Ibuprofen

_____ Docusate sodium

_____ Oxycodone

_____ Acetaminophen

→ • Click on **Return to Room 503**.
  • Click on the **Drug** icon and review the information for acetaminophen.

13. How will acetaminophen reduce Kathryn Doyle's temperature?

14. How soon should Kathryn Doyle's temperature be retaken once she is given acetaminophen? Why?

15. Identify two nursing diagnoses that would be applicable to Kathryn Doyle's health status and her abnormal vital signs.

Care of the Surgical Wound

 Reading Assignment: Surgical Wound Care (Chapter 13)

Patient: Kathryn Doyle, Room 503 (Disk 1)

Objectives:

1. Define key terms associated with impaired wound healing.
2. Develop nursing diagnoses appropriate for the postoperative patient.
3. Discuss the phases of wound healing.
4. Identify potential complications related to wound healing.

Exercise 1

 Writing Activity

15 minutes

1. Match each of the following phases of wound healing with its correct definition.

Phase of Wound Healing	Definition
_____ Maturation	a. New cells are produced to fill the wound. This process closes the wound and aids in prevention of wound contamination.
_____ Hemostasis	
_____ Reconstruction	b. Fibroblasts exit the wound and the wound continues to gain strength.
_____ Inflammatory	c. Collagen is formed and the wound begins to develop a scar.
	d. This phase begins at the time of the surgery. Blood products adhere to the site of the wound and begin to reduce blood loss.

2. There are several types of wound drainage. For each description of drainage given below, enter the type of fluid associated with it. (*Hint:* See Table 13-2 in your textbook.)

   a. Clear, watery fluid: _____

   b. Drainage containing blood: _____

   c. Thin, watery drainage containing blood: _____

   d. Thick, yellow, green, tan, or brown: _____

3. Match each of the following terms associated with wound complications with its appropriate definition.

Terms	Definition
_____ Abscess	a. Passage of escape into the tissues, usually of blood, serum, or lymph
_____ Adhesion	b. Infection of the skin characterized by heat, pain, erythema, and edema
_____ Cellulitis	
_____ Dehiscence	c. Collection of extravasated blood trapped in the tissues or in an organ resulting from incomplete hemostasis after surgery
_____ Evisceration	
_____ Extravasation	d. Cavity containing pus and surrounded by inflamed tissue, formed as a result of suppuration in a localized infection
_____ Hematoma	
	e. Protrusion of an internal organ through a wound or surgical incision
	f. Band of scar tissue that binds together two anatomic surfaces normally separated; most commonly found in the abdomen
	g. Separation of a surgical incision or rupture of a wound closure

4. Identify the three most common wound complications.

5. What physical findings at a wound site would indicate impaired healing?

6. _____ The majority of wound infections are evident by the time of discharge. (True or False)

7. List several patient factors that may affect wound healing of a postoperative patient.

Exercise 2

CD-ROM Activity

45 minutes

- Using the *Virtual Clinical Excursions—Skilled Nursing* CD (Disk 1), sign in to work at Pacific View Regional Hospital for Period of Care 1. (*Note:* If you are already in the virtual hospital from a previous exercise, click on **Leave the Floor** and **Restart the Program** to get to the sign-in window.)
- From the Patient List, select Kathryn Doyle (Room 503).
- Click on **Get Report** and read the Clinical Report.
- Click on **Go to Nurses' Station** and then on **Chart**.
- Click on **503** to view Kathryn Doyle's chart.
- Click on the **Nursing Admission** tab and review the notes.

1. What was the reason for Kathryn Doyle's admission?

2. What surgical procedure did Kathryn Doyle undergo?

➔ • Click on the **History and Physical** tab and review the report.

3. What complications have necessitated Kathryn Doyle's continued hospitalization?

➔ • Click on **Return to Room 503**.
   • Click on **Patient Care** and complete a head-to-toe physical assessment.

4. Discuss the findings most pertinent to Kathryn Doyle's postoperative recovery.

5. What patient factors are most likely affecting Kathryn Doyle's prolonged recovery? (*Hint:* See Exercise 1, question 7, in this lesson.)

6. What environmental/hospital factors may affect Kathryn Doyle's recovery?

7. Kathryn Doyle's wound does not have a dressing. What is the rationale for allowing the wound to be open to the air?

8. _____ Leaving Kathryn Doyle's wound open to air will increase her risk for infection at the site. (True or False)

9. As discussed earlier, the wound may have drainage during the early postoperative period. What causes this drainage? Does it indicate a problem?

10. Develop three nursing diagnoses for Kathryn Doyle relating to her postoperative period.

11. Develop two positive patient outcomes for Kathryn Doyle.

12. Identify two areas that should be included in the teaching plan for Kathryn Doyle.

13. In addition to the physical assessment, what other assessments should be performed on Kathryn Doyle?

LESSON 8

Pain Management

👓 **Reading Assignment:** Pain Management, Comfort, Rest, and Sleep (Chapter 16)

Patient: Kathryn Doyle, Room 503 (Disk 1)

Objectives:

1. Identify the elements that must be included in an assessment of pain.
2. List medications used in the management of pain.
3. Relate the types/classifications of analgesics with the level of pain they are intended to treat.
4. Provide the appropriate patient education that accompanies the administration of analgesics.

Exercise 1

 Writing Activity

 15 minutes

 1. Identify several behavioral cues that may be associated with the presence of pain. (*Hint:* See Box 16-3 in your textbook.)

2. Identify physiologic signs that may be associated with the presence of pain. (*Hint:* See Box 16-3 in your textbook.)

3. For what types of pain are nonopioids usually prescribed?

4. For what types of pain are opioids normally prescribed?

5. What should the nurse tell a patient who voices concerns about becoming addicted to opioid-containing medications?

6. The _____ is a battery-operated device that provides a continuous mild electrical current and blocks pain impulses.

7. Indicate whether each of the following statements is true or false.

   a. _____ The risk for gastric toxicity from NSAIDs is greater in older adults.

   b. _____ The treatment of pain in the older adult is as likely to be successful as that in a younger person.

8. Which of the following is associated with the undertreatment of pain by health care providers?

_____ Concerns about the cost of medications prescribed

_____ Inadequate information about the drugs ordered

_____ Anxiety about potential patient injuries suffered while being medicated

_____ Laziness of the health care provider

_____ Concerns about fostering an addiction

_____ Safety issues

9. _____ is felt at a site other than the injured or diseased organ or part of the body.

Exercise 2

 CD-ROM Activity

 45 minutes

- Using the *Virtual Clinical Excursions—Skilled Nursing* CD (Disk 1), sign in to work at Pacific View Regional Hospital for Period of Care 1. (*Note:* If you are already in the virtual hospital from a previous exercise, click on **Leave the Floor** and **Restart the Program** to get to the sign-in window.)
- From the Patient List, select Kathryn Doyle (Room 503).
- Click on **Get Report** and read the Clinical Report.
- Click on **Go to Nurses' Station** and then on **503** to enter the patient's room.
- Read the Initial Observation notes.
- Click on **Take Vital Signs**.

1. How does Kathryn Doyle describe her pain?

 • Click on **Chart** and then on **503** to view Kathryn Doyle's chart.
- Click the **History and Physical** tab and review the report.

2. Review the reason for Kathryn Doyle's continued hospitalization.

• Click on **Return to Room 503**.
   • Click on **MAR** and then on tab **503** to view Kathryn Doyle's Medication Administration
     Record.
   • Review the medications prescribed.
   • Click on the **Drug** icon as needed to review the drug resource guide.

3. Which of the following medications have been prescribed for Kathryn Doyle to help reduce
   her pain?

   _____ Calcium citrate

   _____ Oxycodone

   _____ Ibuprofen

   _____ Ferrous sulfate

   _____ Docusate sodium

   _____ Acetaminophen

4. How are each of the above medications ordered for Kathryn Doyle (scheduled or prn)?
   Why?

5. Identify the classifications of each of the medications reviewed in questions 3 and 4.

6. What special considerations should be evaluated when administering pain medications to
   Kathryn Doyle?

7. Which of the following best explains the rationale for ibuprofen being prescribed on a scheduled basis rather than prn?
   a. Ibuprofen can also reduce the risk for infection and can be beneficial to the postoperative patient.
   b. Ibuprofen has antiinflammatory properties, which aid the surgical patient in the recovery process.
   c. Ibuprofen is stronger than the other ordered analgesic medications and is more necessary to her recovery.
   d. The scheduling of ibuprofen on a set schedule will help to keep her temperature reduced.

8. When administering oxycodone, the nurse should anticipate which of the following side effects? Select all that apply.

   _____   Drowsiness

   _____   Nervousness

   _____   Agitation

   _____   Hypotension

   _____   Tachycardia

   _____   Anorexia

9. What should be assessed prior to the administration of oxycodone?

10. What patient education should be provided to Kathryn Doyle concerning oxycodone?

11. _____   If Kathryn Doyle reports having difficulty swallowing the oxycodone tablets, encouraging her to chew them is acceptable practice.
    (True or False)

12. In addition to medication therapy, what nursing interventions may be implemented to reduce her level of pain?

13. _____ Kathryn Doyle is suffering from chronic pain. (True or False)

LESSON **9** ───────────────────────────

Patient Safety

────────────────────────────────────

 Reading Assignment: Safety (Chapter 14)

Patient: Kathryn Doyle, Room 503 (Disk 1)

Objectives:

1. Discuss safety factors related to advancing age.
2. Identify factors related to hospitalization that increase the risk for falls.
3. Discuss nursing interventions that reduce the safety risk of the hospitalized patient.
4. Develop nursing diagnoses related to patient safety.

Exercise 1

 Writing Activity

15 minutes

1. When employing the use of a gait belt to assist with ambulation, which of the following are appropriate techniques? Select all that apply.

   _____ The gait belt should fit loosely around the hips.

   _____ The gait belt should be removed or loosened after use.

   _____ Walk behind the patient with the belt in hand to prevent falls.

   _____ Walk beside the patient with one arm around the waist and the other hand on the belt.

2. What risk factors increase with age?

3. List several physiologic changes that may contribute to older adults' risk for injury. (*Hint:* See page 352 in your textbook.)

4. What variables associated with hospitalization may increase a patient's risk for falls?

5. Indicate whether each of the following statements is true or false.

   a. _____ Nurses should use restraint devices whenever a patient is at risk for falls.

   b. _____ Special interventions should be implemented to accommodate a left-handed patient.

6. The national organization that provides guidelines to help reduce safety hazards in the

   workplace is called the _____.

Exercise 2

 CD-ROM Activity

 45 minutes

- Using the *Virtual Clinical Excursions—Skilled Nursing* CD (Disk 1), sign in to work at Pacific View Regional Hospital for Period of Care 2. (*Note:* If you are already in the virtual hospital from a previous exercise, click on **Leave the Floor** and **Restart the Program** to get to the sign-in window.)
- From the Patient List, select Kathryn Doyle (Room 503).
- Click on **Get Report** and read the Clinical Report.
- Click on **Go to Nurses' Station** and then on **503** to enter the patient's room.
- Read the Initial Observation notes.
- Click on **Check Armband** and then on **Take Vital Signs**.
- Click on **Patient Care** and perform a head-to-toe assessment of Kathryn Doyle.

1. What factors listed on Kathryn Doyle's armband are indicative of a safety risk factor?

2. When performing an environmental assessment for Kathryn Doyle, the nurse should include which of the following factors?

_____ Pathways to the bathroom, door, and closet

_____ Patient's emotional well-being

_____ Availability of operational call light

_____ Family's understanding of the plan of care

_____ Patient's knowledge of the unit routine

3. What findings in Kathryn Doyle's physical assessment may increase her risk for falls?

4. Describe the nursing interventions that should be implemented to compensate for Kathryn Doyle's impairments listed in your answer to question 3. Give a rationale for each.

5. When assessing safety risk, the patient's physical assessment, laboratory results, physical

   health history, and _____ should be taken into account.

→ • Click on **MAR** and review Kathryn Doyle's prescribed medications.

6. Which of the following prescribed medications may increase the patient's safety risk? Select all that apply.

   _____ Acetaminophen

   _____ Oxycodone

   _____ Ibuprofen

   _____ Ferrous sulfate

   _____ Calcium citrate

7. If the medications discussed in the previous question are administered, what special precautions should be initiated?

8. Medications that can pose safety risks for older adult patients include which of the following? Select all that apply.

   _____ Vitamins

   _____ Diuretics

   _____ Hypnotics

   _____ Antibiotics

   _____ Antihistamines

➜ • Click on **Return to Room 503**.
  • Click on **Chart** and then on **503** to view Kathryn Doyle's chart.
  • Click on and review the **Laboratory Reports** and **Diagnostic Reports** sections.

  9. Have any tests been performed that may provide information concerning the safety risks for Kathryn Doyle?

➜ • Click on the **History and Physical** and review the data given.

  10. What health history information given may be used to assess Kathryn Doyle's safety risks?

  11. When is the use of safety reminder devices (SRDs) indicated?

  12. _____ It is appropriate to use a safety reminder device (SRD) to restrain an extremity for IV therapy. (True or False)

  13. What complications may arise with the use of SRDs?

14. To avoid complications when using SRDs, what interventions should be employed?

15. List techniques that may be used to avoid the use of SRDs.

16. Develop two nursing diagnoses relating to safety for Kathryn Doyle.

Patient Mobility

──

Reading Assignment: Body Mechanics and Patient Mobility (Chapter 15)

Patient: Kathryn Doyle, Room 503 (Disk 1)

Objectives:

1. List the complications associated with immobility.
2. Identify the responsibilities of the nurse concerning documentation of patient ambulation activities.
3. Develop nursing diagnoses for the patient faced with mobility concerns.
4. Discuss the use of range of motion exercises.

Exercise 1

Writing Activity

15 minutes

  1. When a patient with immobility concerns ambulates, what should the nurse monitor and document?

2. Identify common complications associated with immobility. (*Hint:* See Box 15-2 in your textbook.)

3. What patient conditions should be assessed prior to ambulation?

4. Match the following columns to show the correct sequence of steps that must be taken when assisting a patient who faints or collapses during ambulation.

_____ Call for assistance	a. First
_____ Document the event	b. Second
_____ Stand with feet apart and back straight	c. Third
_____ Assist the patient back to bed	d. Fourth
_____ Quickly bring the patient close to your body	e. Fifth
_____ Lower the patient to the floor	f. Sixth

5. Match each of the following positions with its correct definition.

Position		**Definition**
_____	Semi-Fowler's	a. Lying with the head lowered and the body and legs on an incline plane
_____	Orthopneic	
		b. Lying on the back with the head of the bed elevated approximately 30 degrees
_____	Sims'	
_____	Prone	c. Kneeling with the body weight supported by the knees and chest
_____	Lithotomy	
		d. Lying face-down in a horizontal position
_____	Trendelenburg	
		e. Side-lying with the knee and thigh drawn upward toward the chest
_____	Genupectoral	
		f. Sitting up at a 90-degree angle; may be supported by a pillow on the overbed table
		g. Lying supine with hips and knees flexed; thighs abducted and rotated externally

6. What are range-of-motion exercises? Who is responsible for performing them?

7. Match each of the following range-of-motion movements with its correct definition.

Movement		**Definition**
_____	Circumduction	a. Movement of the foot with the toes pointed upward
_____	External rotation	b. Movement of an extremity toward the midline of the body
_____	Dorsiflexion	
		c. Turning of the foot and leg away from the other leg
_____	Adduction	
		d. Movement of an extremity away from the midline of the body
_____	Abduction	
		e. Movement of the arm or leg in a full circle

8. _____ Sunlight influences the rate of bone loss. (True or False)

Exercise 2

 CD-ROM Activity

 45 minutes

- Using the *Virtual Clinical Excursions—Skilled Nursing* CD (Disk 1), sign in to work at Pacific View Regional Hospital for Period of Care 2. (*Note:* If you are already in the Virtual Hospital from a previous exercise, click on **Leave the Floor** and **Restart the Program** to get to the sign-in window.)
- From the Patient List, select Kathryn Doyle (Room 503).
- Click on **Get Report** and read the Clinical Report.
- Click on **Go to Nurses' Station** and then on **Chart**.
- Click on **503** to view Kathryn Doyle's chart.
- Click on the following tabs and review the records: **History and Physical**, **Nursing Admission**, **Physician's Notes**, and **Physician's Orders**.

1. What is Kathryn Doyle's primary medical diagnosis?

2. List Kathryn Doyle's other medical concerns.

3. What activity orders have been made by the physician?

• Click on **Return to Nurses' Station** and then on **503** to go to the patient's room.
  • Read the Initial Observation notes.
  • Click on **Take Vital Signs** and review the information given.
  • Click on **Patient Care** and perform a head-to-toe assessment.

4. When Kathryn Doyle is faced with getting up and ambulating to the dining room, how does she respond?

5. What factors in Kathryn Doyle's medical history may be further complicated by her continued immobility?

6. Based on the assessment, are there any physiologic reasons that Kathryn Doyle is unable to ambulate?

7. Given Kathryn Doyle's refusal to ambulate and the physician's orders requiring her to do so, what should the nurse do?

8. Kathryn Doyle should be repositioned every _____ hours.

9. Kathryn Doyle has a wedge-shaped pillow between her legs. What purpose does this serve?

10. Based on the assessment, is Kathryn Doyle experiencing any of the above complications associated with immobility?

→ • Click on **Chart** and then on **503** to view Kathryn Doyle's chart.
   • Click the **Consultations** tab and review the information given.

11. What consultations have been made to improve/increase Kathryn Doyle's mobility?

12. What assistive devices have been employed for the patient to increase her mobility? What is the purpose of these devices?

13. Which of the following actions are the nurse's responsibility concerning Kathryn Doyle's assistive devices? Select all that apply.

_____ The nurse should should perform an assessment to determine whether the assistive devices are being appropriately used.

_____ The nurse should remove the assistive devices for small periods each day to increase the patient's independence.

_____ The nurse must be present whenever the patient uses the assistive devices.

_____ The patient's permanent record must have evidence of the factors selected above.

_____ The patient should be taught the appropriate use of the devices.

_____ The devices should be evaluated to ensure they are in working order.

14. In physical therapy, how much assistance is needed for Kathryn Doyle's ambulation?

15. What is being done in the physical therapy department to increase the physical strength of her lower body?

16. What special considerations are needed for Kathryn Doyle with regard to range-of-motion exercises because of her age?

17. In addition to the ROM exercises, what other treatments/activities are being done by the physical therapy department?

18. Develop two nursing diagnoses relating to Kathryn Doyle's mobility status.

LESSON **11** ————————————————————

Nutritional Assessment in a Malnourished Patient

————————————————————————————————

Ꝺ **Reading Assignment:** Basic Nutrition and Nutritional Therapy (Chapter 21)

Patient: Kathryn Doyle, Room 503 (Disk 1)

Objectives:

1. Identify effects of nutritional status on postoperative recovery.
2. Define osteoporosis.
3. List the risk factors associated with the development of osteoporosis.
4. Discuss the role of the nurse in the promotion of healthy nutrition.

Exercise 1

 Writing Activity

 15 minutes

1. What is osteoporosis? What effects does this disorder have on the body?

2. Which of the following factors contribute to the development of osteoporosis? Select all that apply.

_____ Genetic influences

_____ Physical activity

_____ Gender

_____ Large skeletal frame

_____ Reduced intake of vitamin D, fluoride, and other trace minerals

_____ Menopause

_____ Smoking

3. Match each dietary nutrient with its correct definition.

Nutrient	**Definition**
_____ Complete proteins	a. Substances of plant origin which lack one or more of the essential amino acids
_____ Incomplete proteins	b. Organic compounds essential in small quantities for normal physiologic and metabolic functioning of the body
_____ Vitamins	
_____ Minerals	c. Inorganic compounds essential in small quantities for normal physiologic and metabolic functioning of the body
_____ Carbohydrates	d. Substances that are generally animal in nature and contain all nine essential amino acids
	e. Energy-producing organic compounds

4. Complete the following list to describe the roles of the nurse in the promotion of healthy nutrition. (*Hint:* See page 611 in your textbook.)

• Providing education to the patient regarding the importance of diet

• Encouraging dietary _____

• Assisting with eating as needed

• Serving meal trays to patients in a _____ and _____ manner

• Measuring the patient's height and weight

• Recording patient _____ and _____

• Observing and reporting clinical signs of _____

• Serving as a _____ among the patient, dietitian, physician, and other members of the health care team

5. List several foods that are good dietary sources of calcium.

6. Identify some dietary factors that will reduce calcium loss in the urine (enter either "Low" or "High").

   • _____-sodium diets

   • _____-potassium diets

   • _____-protein diets

7. Which of the following statements concerning ferrous sulfate are true and should be told to patients taking this medication? Select all that apply.

   _____ Stools will darken in color.

   _____ Stools may appear clay-colored.

   _____ Take the medication on an empty stomach to avoid nausea.

   _____ Take the medication after meals or with food if GI discomforts occur.

   _____ Do not take within 2 hours of antacids.

   _____ Do not take the medication with milk or eggs.

   _____ This medication may reduce the effectiveness of some antibiotics.

8. List several foods that are good dietary sources of iron.

9. Which factors can inhibit iron absorption? Select all that apply. (*Hint:* See Box 21-4 in your textbook.)

_____ Some medications, such as antacids

_____ Fish, meat, and poultry containing MFP

_____ Calcium in milk and supplements

_____ Polyphenols, compounds found in coffee, tea, and red wine

_____ Ascorbic acid (vitamin C) when ingested with iron-containing foods

10. _____ Nonheme iron is well-absorbed from the GI tract. (True or False)

11. How do complete and incomplete proteins differ?

Exercise 2

 CD-ROM Activity

 45 minutes

- Using the *Virtual Clinical Excursions—Skilled Nursing* CD (Disk 1), sign in to work at Pacific View Regional Hospital for Period of Care 3. (*Note:* If you are already in the virtual hospital from a previous exercise, click on **Leave the Floor** and **Restart the Program** to get to the sign-in window.)
- From the Patient List, select Kathryn Doyle (Room 503).
- Click on **Get Report** and read the Clinical Report.
- Click on **Go to Nurses' Station** and then on **503** to enter the patient's room.
- Read the Initial Observation notes.
- Click on **Chart** and then on **503** to view Kathryn Doyle's chart.
- Click on the following tabs and review these records: **History and Physical**, **Nursing Admission**, and **Consultations**.

1. What complications of Kathryn Doyle's surgery are reported in the History and Physical?

2. According to the Consultations, what is the physician's impression concerning the nutritional status of this patient?

3. Which of the postoperative complications identified in question 1 of this exercise are further complicated by Kathryn Doyle's nutritional status? Why does her nutritional status have these effects?

4. What risk factors for the development of osteoporosis does Kathryn Doyle have?

5. Kathryn Doyle reports that she has lost 4 pounds in the last 5 months (15 pounds in the last 2 years). What psychosocial factors may have contributed to her weight loss?

6. What is one physical factor that may have contributed to her weight loss?

7. What are the impressions of the dietary consultation?

8. Discuss the plan outlined in the dietary consultation.

9. What is the purpose of the dietary supplements that have been ordered for Kathryn Doyle?

10. What role will the increased protein have in her diet?

11. Which foods are excluded in a soft diet? (*Hint:* See pages 636-637 in your textbook.)

 • Click on **Physician's Orders** and review the information given.

12. What medications have been ordered to aid Kathryn Doyle in meeting the nutritional requirements of her body and health status?

 • Click on **Return to Room 503**.
• Click on the **Drug** icon and review the medications you identified in question 12.

13. What nursing considerations should be observed when administering each of these drugs?

 • Click **Return to Room 503**.
• Read the Initial Observation notes.
• Click on **Take Vital Signs** and review the information given.
• Click on **Patient Care** and perform a head-to-toe physical assessment.

14. What assessment findings are related to Kathryn Doyle's limited nutritional intake?

15. What dietary nutrients would aid Kathryn Doyle in increasing her energy level?

16. What positive effects will an increase in fluid intake have on Kathryn Doyle's assessment findings?

17. To ensure that Kathryn Doyle meets the increased fluid intake order, what should the nurse do?

18. If Kathryn Doyle refuses to increase her intake, what noninvasive measures can the nurse take?

Nutritional Assessment in an Overweight Patient

 Reading Assignment: Basic Nutrition and Nutritional Therapy (Chapter 21)

Patient: Delores Gallegos, Room 502 (Disk 1)

Objectives:

1. Identify the health risks that accompany obesity.
2. Calculate the caloric needs of a patient.
3. Discuss the impact of aging on caloric needs.
4. Discuss the relationship between diuretic therapy and nutritional needs.

Exercise 1

 Writing Activity

🕐 30 minutes

1. How is obesity defined?

2. How is obesity measured? Using this measurement method, what is considered obese?

3. List several health risks associated with obesity. (*Hint:* See page 638 in your textbook.)

4. What treatments are available for the treatment of obesity?

5. Match each of the following foods with the fatty acid class to which it belongs.

Food	Fatty Acid Class
_____ Margarine	a. Saturated
_____ Corn oil	b. Monounsaturated
_____ Beef tallow	c. Polyunsaturated
_____ Egg yolk	d. Trans
_____ Coconut oil	
_____ Chicken fat	
_____ Most fish oils	
_____ Peanuts	
_____ Olives	

6. Potassium has several functions in the human body. Complete the following list describing the actions of potassium.

   • Helps to regulate _____ and _____ within cells

   • Promotes transmission of _____ impulses

   • Aids in functioning of _____ muscles

   • Assists in the regulation of _____ balance

7. What clinical manifestations are associated with low levels of potassium?

8. Which of the following are considered good sources of dietary potassium? Select all that apply.

   _____ Fruits

   _____ Leafy green vegetables

   _____ Avocados

   _____ Legumes

   _____ Nuts

   _____ Milk

   _____ Potatoes

9. The feeling of fullness and satisfaction from ingestion of food is known as

   _____.

Exercise 2

 CD-ROM Activity

 30 minutes

- Using the *Virtual Clinical Excursions—Skilled Nursing* CD (Disk 1), sign in to work at Pacific View Regional Hospital for Period of Care 1. (*Note:* If you are already in the virtual hospital from a previous exercise, click on **Leave the Floor** and **Restart the Program** to get to the sign-in window.)
- From the Patient List, select Delores Gallegos (Room 502).
- Click on **Get Report** and read the Clinical Report.
- Click on **Go to Nurses' Station** and then on **Chart**.
- Click on **502** to view Delores Gallegos' chart.
- Click on the following tabs and review these records: **History and Physical**, **Physician's Notes**, **Physician's Orders**, and **Nursing Admission**.

1. According to the patient's physical exam, how is Delores Gallegos' weight described?

2. In what manner has Delores Gallegos' weight affected her health status?

3. What other significant health history is identified?

➤ • Click on **Return to Nurses' Station** and then on **MAR**.
 • Click on tab **502** to view Delores Gallegos' MAR.

4. The following medications have been ordered for Delores Gallegos to treat her heart failure. Match each medication with its intended effect.

Medication	**Mechanism of Action**
_____ Furosemide	a. Slows heart rate; decreases blood pressure and cardiac output
_____ Captopril	b. Produces a diuretic effect
_____ Metoprolol	c. Improves cardiac output and increases exercise tolerance

5. Why do electrolyte disturbances occur with the administration of furosemide?

6. What laboratory functions should be monitored with diuretic therapy?

➤ • Click on **Return to Nurses' Station**.
 • Click on **Chart** and then on **502** to view Delores Gallegos' chart.
 • Click on **Laboratory Reports** and review the results provided.

7. The normal value for potassium within the body is between _____ and _____ mEq/L.

8. How do Delores Gallegos' electrolytes in the laboratory results for Wednesday at 0600 compare with normal limits?

→ • Click on **Return to Nurses' Station** and then on **502** to go to the patient's room.
  • Click on **Patient Care** and then on **Nurse-Client Interactions**.
  • Select and view the video titled **0730: Cultural Preferences**. (*Note:* Check the virtual clock to see whether enough time has elapsed. You can use the fast-forward feature to advance the time by 2-minute intervals if the video is not yet available. Then click on **Patient Care** and **Nurse-Client Interactions** to refresh the screen.)

9. What is Delores Gallegos' chief complaint regarding her hospital diet?

10. What are the responsibilities of the nurse when faced with concerns such as those of Delores Gallegos?

11. How does culture affect dietary intake?

→ • Click on **Check Armband** and review the information given.

12. What impact does Delores Gallegos' age have on her caloric needs?

13. How would you approximate the patient's caloric needs?

14. The dietary consultation is pending. What dietary recommendations would you anticipate for Delores Gallegos?

LESSON **13** —————————————————————————

Basic Mental Health Nursing Concepts

———————————————————————————————————————

Reading Assignment: Basic Concepts of Mental Health (Chapter 34)

Patient: Carlos Reyes, Room 504 (Disk 1)

Objectives:

1. Discuss the evaluation of mental health along a continuum.
2. Identify factors that affect a patient's position on the mental health continuum.
3. Discuss the impact of hospitalization on mental health.
4. Discuss nursing interventions to reduce the stressors associated with hospitalization.

Exercise 1

 Writing Activity

 15 minutes

1. How is mental health defined?

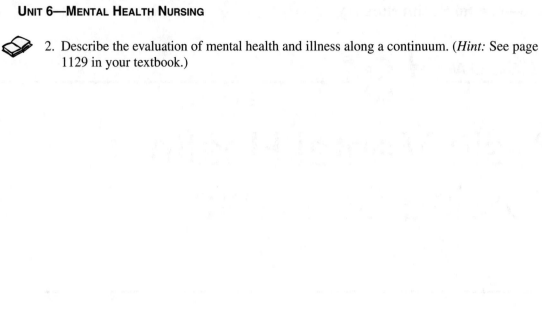

2. Describe the evaluation of mental health and illness along a continuum. (*Hint:* See page 1129 in your textbook.)

3. What factors must be assessed to determine a patient's placement along the continuum?

4. Mental illness may be characterized by patterns of behavior that are _____,

_____, or _____.

5. _____ Defense mechanisms are inadequate behaviors used to protect the personality in times of stress. (True or False)

6. Match each commonly used defense mechanism with its correct description. (*Hint:* See Table 34-1 in your textbook.)

Defense mechanism	**Description**
_____ Compensation	a. An avoidance of reality
_____ Conversion	b. The intentional exclusion of painful thoughts, experiences, or impulses
_____ Denial	c. Excelling in one area to make up for deficits in another area
_____ Displacement	
_____ Identification	d. Placing the blame for personal shortcomings on another person or group
_____ Projection	e. Turing emotional conflicts into a physical symptom
_____ Rationalization	f. A process of making plausible reasons to justify or explain one's behavior
_____ Suppression	g. An individual's incorporation of a characteristic belonging to another person or group
	h. The expression of emotions toward someone or something other than the source of the emotion

7. What is meant by the term "flat affect"?

8. List several factors associated with the hospital environment that may have an impact on the mental health of a patient who has been hospitalized.

9. Indicate whether each of the following is true or false.

a. _____ Reminiscence and life review are ineffective techniques to help the older adult successfully cope with changing life circumstances.

b. _____ Older people experiencing sensory changes may have behavioral changes that could be mistaken for disorientation.

Exercise 2

 CD-ROM Activity

 45 minutes

- Using the *Virtual Clinical Excursions—Skilled Nursing* CD (Disk 1), sign in to work at Pacific View Regional Hospital for Period of Care 1. (*Note:* If you are already in the virtual hospital from a previous exercise, click on **Leave the Floor** and then **Restart the Program** to get to the sign-in window.)
- From the Patient List, select Carlos Reyes (Room 504).
- Click on **Get Report** and read the Clinical Report.
- Click on **Go to Nurse's Station** and then on **Chart**. Click on **504** to view Carlos Reyes' chart.
- Review the **History and Physical** and **Nursing Admission** sections of the chart.

1. Why is Carlos Reyes being transferred to the Skilled Nursing Unit?

2. List significant factors recorded in Carlos Reyes' past medical history.

3. Describe Carlos Reyes' demeanor during the admission nursing assessment.

4. Identify factors that may influence the amount and/or degree of anxiety that Carlos Reyes may experience.

5. What does Carlos Reyes' family report concerning his cognitive status?

 • Click on **Return to Nurses' Station** and then on **504** to enter the patient's room.
 • Read the Initial Observation notes.
 • Next, click on **Take Vital Signs** and review the information given.
 • Also click on and read the **Clinical Alerts**.
 • Now click on **Patient Care** and perform a head-to-toe assessment.

6. List any mental health abnormalities noted during the assessment of Carlos Reyes.

7. What sensory changes associated with aging may further affect Carlos Reyes' ability to respond appropriately to environmental stimuli?

8. What other factors associated with aging may impact Carlos Reyes' mental health?

9. What impact might Carlos Reyes' myocardial infarction have on his mental health?

10. Which of the following factors will affect the level of anxiety that Carlos Reyes may experience in response to the stressors he is encountering? Select all that apply.

_____ How the patient views the stressors

_____ The number of stressors being managed at the same time

_____ The perception of stress by his health care team

_____ Past experience with similar situations

_____ The degree of significance the stressor will have on his future

11. Identify nursing interventions to reduce the stressors associated with Carlos Reyes' hospitalization.

 • Click on **Patient Care** and then on **Nurse-Client Interactions**.
 • Select and view the video titled **0740: Family Teaching—Medication**. (*Note:* Check the virtual clock to see whether enough time has elapsed. You can use the fast-forward feature to advance the time by 2-minute intervals if the video is not yet available. Then click on **Patient Care** and **Nurse-Client Interactions** to refresh the screen.)

12. Describe Carlos Reyes' level of responsiveness during the video interaction.

13. What concerns are being voiced by Carlos Reyes' son?

14. The nurse tells Carlos Reyes' son that his father has been given a medication called

    _____.

→ • Click on **Chart** and then on **504** to view Carlos Reyes' chart.
  • Click on the **Nurse's Notes** tab and review the information given.

15. In addition to the medication prescribed for Carlos Reyes, what other factors may be contributing to his level of responsiveness?

→ • Click on **Return to Room 504**.
  • Click on the **Drug** icon and review the information for the drug that Carlos Reyes has been given.

16. Which of the following are indications for the administration of this medication? Select all that apply.

    _____ Pain

    _____ Intermittent confusion

    _____ Mild to moderate anxiety

    _____ Severe anxiety

    _____ Hallucinations

    _____ Alcohol withdrawal

17. What side effects may be encountered with the administration of this medication?

18. What safety interventions and/or precautions should be implemented for patients taking this drug?

19. What actions have been taken by the nurse in response to the family's concerns and the patient's condition?

Care of the Patient with a Psychiatric Disorder

 Reading Assignment: Care of the Patient with a Psychiatric Disorder (Chapter 35)

Patient: Carlos Reyes, Room 504 (Disk 1)

Objectives:

1. Identify abnormal findings related to mental health status during a physical assessment.
2. Identify nonverbal cues in the nurse-patient interaction.
3. List nursing interventions to promote and/or develop therapeutic communication.
4. Define the various types of anxiety disorders.
5. List defense mechanisms that may be used by the patient experiencing stress.

Exercise 1

 Writing Activity

 30 minutes

1. Numerous techniques may be used in psychiatric therapy. Match each therapeutic technique with its correct description. (*Hint:* See page 1154 in your textbook.)

Therapeutic Technique	Description
_____ Behavior therapy	a. The use of toys and puppets to express feelings
_____ Cognitive therapy	b. Used to relieve anxiety by conditioning and retraining responses by repetition
_____ Group therapy	
_____ Play therapy	c. A long-term process used to bring unconscious feelings to the surface
_____ Free association	d. Breaking negative thought patterns and developing positive feelings about memories or thoughts
_____ Psychoanalysis	e. The joining of patients sharing similar concerns and experiences
	f. Speaking thoughts without censorship

131

2. What is dementia?

3. What type of dementia is seen most commonly in the United States?

4. Two key elements in the nursing care of patients with dementia are providing a

_____ and using _____
techniques.

5. What is caregiver strain?

6. Which of the following statements concerning sundowning syndrome is correct?
   a. Sundowning syndrome often begins in early adulthood and is characterized by a lack of energy in the evening hours.
   b. Sundowning syndrome involves an increase in disorientation in the evening hours.
   c. Schizophrenic patients are at increased risk for developing sundowning syndrome if their medications are interrupted.
   d. Catatonic behavior noted in the evening hours is a clinical manifestation associated with sundowning syndrome.

7. What are generalized anxiety disorders?

8. Match each of the following anxiety disorders with its appropriate definition.

Disorder

_____ Free-floating anxiety

_____ Signal anxiety

_____ Panic attack

_____ Phobia

_____ Obsessive-compulsive disorder

_____ Posttraumatic stress disorder

Definition

a. An irrational fear in which the person dwells on the object of anxiety

b. A response to an intense traumatic experience that is greater than the usual range for normal life events

c. A learned response to an event

d. Recurrent, intrusive thoughts that produce anxiety and repetitive, ritualistic behaviors

e. Feelings of dread that cannot be identified

f. Acute, intense, and overwhelming anxiety accompanied by a degree of personality disorganization and inability to solve problems or think clearly

9. The use of pharmacologic interventions may involve numerous side effects. Match each commonly seen side effect with its correct definition.

Side Effect

_____ Akathisia

_____ Tardive dyskinesia

_____ Dystonias

_____ Dyskinesia

Definition

a. Aberrant posturing

b. Involuntary movements

c. An inability to sit still with continuous movements

d. An extrapyramidal reaction occurring when medication is reduced

10. In addition to medications, what natural or herbal medications may be used in the treatment of mental health conditions?

11. What concerns accompany the use of herbal and natural medications?

Exercise 2

 CD-ROM Activity

 30 minutes

- Using the *Virtual Clinical Excursions—Skilled Nursing* CD (Disk 1), sign in to work at Pacific View Regional Hospital for Period of Care 2. (*Note:* If you are already in the virtual hospital from a previous exercise, click on **Leave the Floor** and **Restart the Program** to get to the sign-in window.)
- From the Patient List, select Carlos Reyes (Room 504).
- Click on **Get Report** and read the Clinical Report.
- Click on **Go to Nurses' Station** and then on **504** to enter the patient's room.
- Click on **Patient Care** and perform a head-to-toe physical assessment.

1. What are the primary concerns for Carlos Reyes reported from the previous shift?

2. Several elements associated with Carlos Reyes' mental health are not within normal limits. According to his physical assessment, how would you describe his:

- Orientation? _____

- Level of consciousness? _____

- Concentration? _____

- Memory? _____

- Speech patterns? _____

- Communication? _____

- Mental state? _____

➤ • Click on **Nurse-Client Interactions**.
- Select and view the video titled **1120: The Agitated Patient**. (*Note:* Check the virtual clock to see whether enough time has elapsed. You can use the fast-forward feature to advance the time by 2-minute intervals if the video is not yet available. Then click on **Patient Care** and **Nurse-Client Interactions** to refresh the screen.)

3. Describe Carlos Reyes' mental status and responses to the nurse's attempt at interaction. Include his nonverbal cues.

4. What interventions can the nurse employ to promote and/or develop therapeutic communication with Carlos Reyes?

→ • Click on **Chart** and then on **504** to view Carlos Reyes' chart.
 • Click on the following tabs and review these records: **Physician's Orders**, **History and Physical**, and **Consultations**.

5. What is the physician's impression of Carlos Reyes' mental health status as reported in the History and Physical?

6. What consultations have been ordered and/or completed?

7. Describe the impressions of the discharge planning coordinator.

8. Who is the primary caregiver for Carlos Reyes?

• Click on **Return to Room 504**.
   • Click on **Patient Care** and then on **Nurse-Client Interactions**.
   • Select and view the videos titled **1140: Assessing for Referrals** and **1145: Intervention—Referral**. (*Note:* Check the virtual clock to see whether enough time has elapsed. You can use the fast-forward feature to advance the time by 2-minute intervals if the video is not yet available. Then click on **Patient Care** and **Nurse-Client Interactions** to refresh the screen.)

9. How does Carlos Reyes' son feel that this hospitalization has affected his father's mental status?

10. Discuss the conflict between the Reyes children.

11. Listed below are medications and dosages prescribed for Carlos Reyes. Match each medication with its intended purpose.

Medication	Intended Purpose
_____ Tacrine 30 mg QID	a. Reduce anxiety
_____ Oxazepam 15 mg TID	b. Increase cognitive functioning
_____ Triazolam 0.125 mg at bedtime	c. Help patient sleep
_____ Lorazepam 0.5 mg PO q12h	

12. Below, identify the possible side effects for each of the medications prescribed for Carlos Reyes.

   • Tacrine: _____

   • Oxazepam: _____

   • Triazolam: _____

   • Lorazepam: _____

LESSON 15 _____

Life Span Development

_____

/O̅D̅ **Reading Assignment:** Life Span Development (Chapter 8)

Patient: Kathryn Doyle, Room 503 (Disk 1)

Objectives:

1. Identify role changes associated with aging.
2. Discuss the developmental tasks associated with older adults.
3. Define physiologic theories associated with aging.
4. Define the psychologic theories associated with aging.

Exercise 1

 Writing Activity

 15 minutes

1. The woman assumes the role of the dominant partner with regard to financial matters, child

   care, and homemaking in the _____ family.

2. Which of the following statements concerning the needs of the aging adult is correct?
   a. Caloric needs will increase only slightly to meet the demands put on the body.
   b. Older adults generally sleep fewer hours per night than they did when they were younger.
   c. The importance of relationships becomes lessened after age 70.
   d. The intensity of sexual drives remains constant throughout the life span.

3. The body's response to aging includes which of the following changes? Select all that apply. (*Hint:* See Table 8-4 in your textbook.)

_____ Body weight increases until age 45 or 50.

_____ The accumulation of adipose tissue in women is more pronounced in the waist, chest, and lower abdomen.

_____ The risk for scoliosis increases in adults between the ages of 50 and 70 years.

_____ Loss of height begins to occur after age 50.

_____ There is a reduction in the perception of taste and smell.

_____ An increase in basal metabolic rate is normal.

4. Indicate whether each of the following statements is true or false.

a. _____ A necessary developmental skill in late adulthood is maximization of independence and maintenance of a high level of involvement.

b. _____ Older people are generally slower than younger people with regard to cognition but often are more accurate.

5. Older adults should maintain a daily fluid intake of _____ mL/day.

6. What are the chief determinants of an individual's psychologic response to aging?

7. The period known as "young older adult" includes people between the ages of _____

and _____.

8. A form of discrimination and prejudice against the older adult is known as

_____.

9. Match each physiologic aging theory with its correct definition. (*Hint:* See pages 180-181 in your textbook.)

Physiologic Aging Theory	**Definition**
_____ Autoimmunity theory	a. Supports the belief that structural and functional changes associated with advancing age are increased by abuses on the body
_____ Free radical theory	
_____ Wear and tear theory	b. Supports the belief that the response to aging is determined by genetic connections
_____ Biologic programming theory	c. Supports the belief that the body is less able to remain free of infection and detrimental processes as it grows older
	d. Supports the belief that an accumulation of cellular waste promotes the aging process

 10. Match each psychologic aging theory with its correct definition. (*Hint:* See page 181 in your textbook.)

Psychologic Aging Theory	**Definition**
_____ Disengagement theory	a. Links successful aging to the ability to maintain roles and activities
_____ Activity theory	
_____ Continuity theory	b. The removal of the aging individual from other elements of society
	c. The belief that interaction with others will promote self-esteem and result in a more positive response to aging

Exercise 2

 CD-ROM Activity

 45 minutes

- Using the *Virtual Clinical Excursions—Skilled Nursing* CD (Disk 1), sign in to work at Pacific View Regional Hospital for Period of Care 3. (*Note:* If you are already in the virtual hospital from a previous exercise, click on **Leave the Floor** and **Restart the Program** to get to the sign-in window.)
- From the Patient List, select Kathryn Doyle (Room 503).
- Click on **Get Report** and read the Clinical Report.
- Click on **Go to Nurses' Station** and then on **503** to enter the patient's room.
- Click on **Check Armband** and review the information given.
- Click on **Chart** and then on **503** to view Kathryn Doyle's chart.
- Click on the following tabs and read these records: **Nursing Admission**, **History and Physical**, and **Consultations**.

1. How old is Kathryn Doyle?

2. What are her primary psychosocial concerns?

3. What does Kathryn Doyle find stressful about her home life?

4. The Doyle household and its inhabitants are an example of a(n) _____ family.

5. Kathryn Doyle is at the _____ stage in the life cycle.

6. Discuss the role changes that Kathryn Doyle has encountered since the death of her spouse.

7. American psychoanalyst Erik Erikson saw the life cycle as a series of

    _____, each of which includes specific tasks or
    challenges.

8. Kathryn Doyle is experiencing the Erikson stage of psychosocial development known as

    _____ versus _____.

9. What takes place during this stage?

10. Based on Kathryn Doyle's responses in the admission assessment, evaluate her success in
    this stage of development.

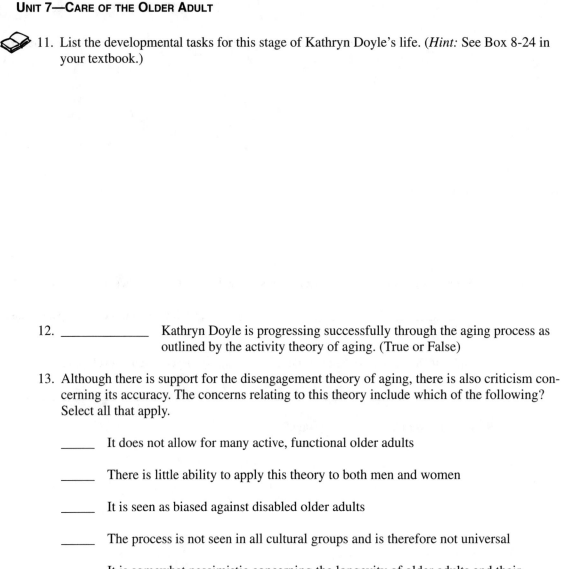 11. List the developmental tasks for this stage of Kathryn Doyle's life. (*Hint:* See Box 8-24 in your textbook.)

12. _____ Kathryn Doyle is progressing successfully through the aging process as outlined by the activity theory of aging. (True or False)

13. Although there is support for the disengagement theory of aging, there is also criticism concerning its accuracy. The concerns relating to this theory include which of the following? Select all that apply.

_____ It does not allow for many active, functional older adults

_____ There is little ability to apply this theory to both men and women

_____ It is seen as biased against disabled older adults

_____ The process is not seen in all cultural groups and is therefore not universal

_____ It is somewhat pessimistic concerning the longevity of older adults and their abilities to continue as contributing members of society

14. According to Erikson, adults who do not find satisfaction with their accomplishments will experience _____ and _____.

15. _____ Some widowed older adults in need of companionship will consider remarrying as a solution to the challenges presented by the death of a spouse. (True or False)

16. Acceptance of one's own _____ and preparation for death are tasks associated with late adulthood.

LESSON 16

Health Promotion in the Older Adult

 Reading Assignment: Health Promotion and Care of the Older Adult (Chapter 33)

Patient: Carlos Reyes, Room 504 (Disk 1)

Objectives:

1. Identify physiologic concerns associated with aging.
2. Identify physiologic changes associated with aging.
3. Identify psychosocial concerns associated with aging.
4. Develop nursing interventions to promote the care of the older adult.

Exercise 1

 Writing Activity

 30 minutes

1. Older adults may face _____ and _____ regarding their changing roles within society and the family.

2. What interventions may be used to increase a patient's orientation to reality? (*Hint:* See page 1114 in your textbook.)

3. The progressive impairment of cognitive function is known as _____.

4. Which of the following integumentary system changes are associated with aging? Select all that apply. (*Hint:* See pages 1094-1095 in your textbook.)

_____ Increased production of sebum

_____ Increased bruising and susceptibility to trauma

_____ Reduction in perspiration

_____ Decreased wound healing time

_____ Increased susceptibility to infection

5. How are urinary and fecal incontinence related to aging?

6. Match each type of incontinence with its correct definition.

Type of incontinence	Definition
_____ Stress urinary incontinence	a. Associated with central nervous system disorders; characterized by involuntary urine loss after a sudden urge to void
_____ Urge urinary incontinence	
_____ Functional urinary incontinence	b. Occurs as a result of inability or unwillingness to toilet because of physical limitations or emotional issues
	c. Involuntary loss of a small amount of urine with increased abdominal pressure

7. Many changes associated with aging take place in the respiratory system, including the following:

• _____ and _____ of the thoracic cage

• Reduced lung _____

• _____ vital capacity

• Reduced number and effectiveness of the lungs' _____

• Reduced air _____ and secretions

8. Many changes associated with aging take place in the cardiovascular system, including the following:

• Loss of structural _____

• _____ and more _____ heart valves

• Decrease in _____ cells and slowed electrical conduction

• Possible decrease in heart rate

• Reduced cardiac _____

• Development of arteriosclerosis

• Increased risk for _____

9. What nursing interventions may be used to reduce cardiovascular complications?

10. According to the American Medical Association, which of the following are classifications of abuse? Select all that apply.

_____ Physical abuse

_____ Psychologic abuse

_____ Behaviors of isolation

_____ Medical abuse

_____ Neglect

_____ Misuse of assets

11. Which of the following statements are true concerning the use of medications in older adults? Select all that apply.

_____ On average, the older adult takes up to seven prescription medications.

_____ Laxatives and vitamin supplements are commonly used medications among older adults.

_____ The average older adult is currently taking two nonprescription medications.

_____ The use of multiple drugs may reduce the therapeutic benefits of the medications taken.

_____ Using more than one pharmacy to fill prescriptions will increase risk factors associated with polypharmacy.

_____ The body's ability to absorb, transport, and eliminate medications is increased with age.

12. _____ Nearly 25% of people 70 years old and older report falls each year. (True or False)

Exercise 2

 CD-ROM Activity

 30 minutes

- Using the *Virtual Clinical Excursions—Skilled Nursing* CD (Disk 1), sign in to work at Pacific View Regional Hospital for Period of Care 1. (*Note:* If you are already in the virtual hospital from a previous exercise, Click on **Leave the Floor** and **Restart the Program** to get to the sign-in window.)
- From the Patient List, select Carlos Reyes (Room 504).
- Click on **Get Report** and read the Clinical Report.
- Click on **Go to Nurses' Station** and then on **504** to enter the patient's room.
- Click on **Check Armband** and then on **Take Vital Signs** and review the information given.
- Click on **Patient Care** and complete a head-to-toe assessment.

1. How old is Carlos Reyes?

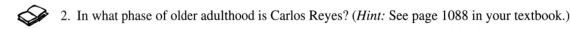 2. In what phase of older adulthood is Carlos Reyes? (*Hint:* See page 1088 in your textbook.)

3. What changes associated with aging are noted in Carlos Reyes' skin and hair?

4. List several abnormalities noted in the head and chest portion Carlos Reyes' physical assessment.

5. Discuss nursing interventions that may be used to compensate for hearing loss.

6. Tackiness of the gums and mucous membranes could be attributed to mild

   _____.

7. List several abnormalities noted in the assessment of Carlos Reyes' upper extremities and abdomen.

8. What impact might nocturia have on Carlos Reyes' health status?

→ • Click on **Chart** and then on **504** to view Carlos Reyes' chart.
  • Click on **History and Physical** and review the information given.

9. Carlos Reyes was admitted to the hospital after experiencing a _____

   _____.

10. Which of the following cardiovascular disease risk factors does Carlos Reyes have? Select all that apply.

    _____ Age

    _____ Lifestyle

    _____ Hyperlipidemia

    _____ Heredity

    _____ Obesity

    _____ Hypertension

11. Does Carlos Reyes have a history of any pulmonary complications and/or disorders?

12. According to the History and Physical, in addition to rehabilitation, why has Carlos Reyes been admitted to the Skilled Nursing Unit?

LESSON **17** ───────────────────────────

Assessment of the Patient with Osteomyelitis

───

 Reading Assignment: Care of the Patient with a Musculoskeletal Disorder
(Chapter 44)

Patient: Harry George, Room 401 (Disk 2)

Objectives:

1. Understand the basic functions of the musculoskeletal system.
2. Review the various types of arthritis.
3. Review risk factors for osteomyelitis.
4. Identify the clinical manifestations of osteomyelitis.
5. Discuss treatment options for the patient with osteomyelitis.

Exercise 1

 Writing Activity

15 minutes

1. The skeletal system serves five major functions:

   a. The skeleton provides the body _____ that supports internal tissues and organs.

   b. The skeleton forms a _____ that protects many internal organs.

   c. Bones provide _____ for movement.

   d. The bones serve as storage areas for various _____.

   e. _____ (blood cell formation) takes place in the red bone marrow.

2. Match each type of body movement with its correct definition. (*Hint:* See Box 44-2 in your textbook.)

**Type of
Body Movement**

_____ Abduction

_____ Adduction

_____ Dorsiflexion

_____ Extension

_____ Flexion

_____ Plantar flexion

_____ Pronation

_____ Rotation

_____ Supination

Definition

a. Movement of the bone around its longitudinal axis.

b. Movement that causes the bottom of the foot to be be directed downward.

c. Movement of certain joints that decreases the angle between two adjoining bones.

d. Movement of the hand and forearm causing the palm to face downward or backward.

e. Movement of an extremity toward the axis of the body.

f. Movement of the hand and forearm that causes the palm to face upward or forward.

g. Movement of certain joints that increases the angle between two adjoining bones.

h. Movement of an extremity away from the midline of the body.

i. Movement that causes the top of the foot to elevate or tilt upward.

3. Which of the following muscles are responsible for movement of the lower extremities? Select all that apply.

_____ Gluteus maximus

_____ Soleus

_____ Masseter

_____ Orbicularis oris

_____ Adductor longus

4. List the four most common types of arthritis.

5. Indicate whether each of the following statements is true or false.

    a. _____ The skeletal muscles are under involuntary control.

    b. _____ Rheumatoid arthritis affects an equal number of men and women.

    c. _____ Children are often diagnosed with osteoarthritis.

6. Osteomyelitis is an infection of bone and/or bone marrow. What are the most common causes of osteomyelitis? (*Hint:* See page 1385 in your textbook.)

7. What is the most common causative agent of osteomyelitis?

8. How is osteomyelitis treated?

Exercise 2

 CD-ROM Activity

 45 minutes

- Using the *Virtual Clinical Excursions—Medical-Surgical* CD (Disk 2), sign in to work at Pacific View Regional Hospital for Period of Care 1. (*Note:* If you are already in the virtual hospital from a previous exercise, click on **Leave the Floor** and then **Restart the Program** to get to the sign-in window.)
- From the Patient List, select Harry George (Room 401).
- Click on **Get Report** and read the Clinical Report.
- Click on **Go to Nurses' Station**; then click on **401** to go to the patient's room.
- Click on **Patient Care** and complete a head-to-toe assessment.

1. When you are assessing Harry George's affected extremity, which factors should you include in the assessment?

2. Harry George was admitted with a diagnosis of osteomyelitis. What findings support this diagnosis?

3. How does the affected extremity appear?

4. How does the assessment of the left (affected) leg differ from that of the right?

5. What other clinical manifestations may accompany a diagnosis of osteomyelitis?

6. How should the affected extremity be positioned?

→ • Click on **Take Vital Signs** and review the information provided.

7. Discuss any findings in Harry George's vital signs that may indicate the presence of infection.

8. Which of the following diagnostic tests may be ordered to support a diagnosis of osteomyelitis? Select all that apply.

_____ MRI

_____ PET scan

_____ Bone scan

_____ X-rays

_____ Serum electrolytes

_____ Erythrocyte sedimentation rate

_____ Blood cultures

_____ Cultures of any drainage from open wounds

_____ Complete blood count

→ • Click on **Chart** and then on **401** to view Harry George's chart.
 • Click on the **Laboratory Reports** and **Diagnostic Reports** tabs and review the information given.

9. What diagnostic tests were ordered for Harry George to support the diagnosis of osteomyelitis?

10. Which lab results support the diagnosis?

11. What findings were reported in the x-ray and bone scan?

→ • Click on the **History and Physical** tab and review the report.

12. Based on your review of Harry George's medical and social history, what risk factors for osteomyelitis does he have?

13. What items in Harry George's assessment will be used to determine effectiveness of treatment?

→ • Click on the **Physician's Orders** tab and review the orders given.

14. What treatments have been ordered to manage Harry George's osteomyelitis?

15. To assist in the management of Harry George's care, what consultations has the physician ordered?

→ • Click on **Return to Room 401**.
 • Click on **MAR** and then on tab **401**. Review the information given.

16. Which of the following medications have been prescribed to treat Harry George's osteomyelitis? Select all that apply.

_____   Gentamicin 20 mg IV

_____   Thiamine 100 mg PO/IM

_____   Glyburide 1.25 mg PO

_____   Cefotaxime 1 g IV

Care of the Patient Experiencing Comorbid Conditions (Musculoskeletal and Endocrine)

Reading Assignment: Care of the Patient with an Endocrine Disorder (Chapter 51)

Patient: Harry George, Room 401 (Disk 2)

Objectives:

1. Describe the functions of the endocrine system.
2. Discuss the dietary limitations of a patient with diabetes.
3. Describe the use of a sliding insulin scale.
4. Explain how type 1 and type 2 diabetes are similar and how they differ.
5. List disorders of the endocrine system.
6. Describe the tests used to assess for the presence of diabetes.

Exercise 1

Writing Activity

 30 minutes

1. The endocrine system functions alongside the _____ system to regulate many functions within the body, including metabolism, growth and development, and reproduction. The endocrine system communicates through the release of

   _____, which are chemical messengers that travel through the bloodstream to their target organs.

2. The _____ is considered the "master gland" of the endocrine system.

3. Match each of the following disorders of the pituitary gland with its correct description.

**Disorder of the
Pituitary Gland**

_____ Acromegaly

_____ Gigantism

_____ Dwarfism

_____ Diabetes insipidus

_____ Syndrome of inappropriate
secretion of antidiuretic
hormone (SIADH)

Description

a. A transient or permanent metabolic disorder of the
posterior pituitary in which ADH is deficient

b. A disorder in which the pituitary gland releases
too much ADH and, in response, the kidneys
reabsorb more water

c. An overproduction of somatotropin in the adult

d. A condition in which there is a deficiency in
growth hormone

e. A condition that usually results from an oversecretion of growth hormone

4. What is diabetes?

 5. How do the two types of diabetes mellitus differ? How are they similar? (*Hint:* See pages
1784-1785 in your textbook.)

6. The exact underlying cause of diabetes is unknown. There are, however, many theories about possible factors that may contribute to the development of diabetes. List several of those factors below.

 7. Match each diagnostic test for diabetes with its function. (*Hint:* See Box 51-2 in your textbook.)

Test	Function
_____ Fasting blood sugar	a. This test is often used to determine whether a patient has type 1 or type 2 diabetes.
_____ Postprandial blood sugar	b. In this test, the fasting patient is provided with a carbohydrate solution to be ingested orally. Two hours after the administration, a blood sample will be drawn.
_____ Glycosylated hemoglobin	
_____ C peptide	c. This test consists of drawing a blood sample after the patient has fasted for an 8-hour period.
	d. This test measures the amount of glucose that has been incorporated into the body's hemoglobin. It reflects the patient's glucose elevations in the past 120 days.

8. Match each type of insulin with its correct onset of action after administration.

Type of Insulin	Onset of Action After Administration
_____ Humalog	a. 15-30 minutes
_____ Regular	b. 30-60 minutes
_____ NPH	c. 1-2 hours
_____ Lente (70/30)	d. 1-3 hours
_____ Lantus	e. 2-4 hours

9. Most available insulin is U/_____.

10. Indicate whether each of the following statements is true or false.

    a. _____ Urine testing is the recommended way of monitoring glucose levels in the IDDM patient.

    b. _____ Lantus should never be mixed with regular insulin.

    c. _____ Diabetics can choose between insulin or oral agents.

11. Insulin should be administered to the _____ tissue.

12. The site with the fastest rate of insulin absorption is the:
    a. abdomen.
    b. arms.
    c. thighs.
    d. buttocks.

13. The loss of fat deposits as a result of insulin administration is known as

_____.

Exercise 2

CD-ROM Activity

30 minutes

- Using the *Virtual Clinical Excursions—Medical-Surgical* CD (Disk 2), sign in to work at Pacific View Regional Hospital for Period of Care 1. (*Note:* If you are already in the virtual hospital from a previous exercise, click on **Leave the Floor** and then **Restart the Program** to get to the sign-in window.)
- From the Patient List, select Harry George (Room 401).
- Click on **Get Report** and read the Clinical Report.
- Click on **Go to Nurses' Station** and then on **Chart**.
- Click on **401** to view Harry George's chart.
- Click on the **Emergency Department** tab and review the information given.

1. What was Harry George's blood glucose upon his arrival at the emergency department?

2. What is the desired blood glucose level for a patient with diabetes?

3. Does Harry George have type 1 or type 2 diabetes mellitus?

4. What medication does Harry George take at home to control his diabetes?

5. How does this type of hypoglycemic medication work?

6. In addition to his daily scheduled medications to control his diabetes, Harry George has a sliding scale. Describe the use of a sliding scale.

7. _____ When Harry George's blood glucose is less than 150 mg/dL, his scheduled oral hypoglycemic medication will be held. (True or False)

8. The blood glucose of an ill patient with diabetes may require monitoring every _____ to

   _____ hours.

9. What impact might illness have on Harry George's blood glucose?

10. How does Harry George's diabetes affect his health status? For which additional complications might he be at risk because of his diabetes?

• Click on **Return to Nurses' Station**; then click on **401** to enter Harry George's room.
• Click on **Patient Care** and then on **Nurse-Client Interactions**.
• Select and view the video titled **0735: Symptom Management**. (*Note:* Check the virtual clock to see whether enough time has elapsed. You can use the fast-forward feature to advance the time by 2-minute intervals if the video is not yet available. Then click on **Patient Care** and **Nurse-Client Interactions** to refresh the screen.)

11. What nonverbal behaviors are displayed by the patient, indicating a problem that needs to be addressed?

12. During the talk between Harry George and his "sitter," what needs and concerns are voiced?

13. What impact does the use of alcohol have on blood glucose level?

 • Click on **Chart** and then on **401** to view Harry George's chart.
• Click on the **Physician's Orders** tab and review the orders.

14. What is the frequency of Harry George's blood glucose assessments?

15. What type of dietary management is being implemented?

16. Which of the following statements concerning Harry George's prescribed diet is correct?
    a. The diet will consist of three full meals per day to prevent snacking.
    b. The fat content should consist of no more than 30% of the caloric intake.
    c. 60% to 70 % of the calories in the diet should be from carbohydrates to ensure energy.
    d. Snacks should be avoided to reduce blood sugar fluctuations.

17. Harry George should be assessed for teaching needed in which areas?

• Click on **Return to Room 401**.
• Click on **Patient Care** and then on **Nurse-Client Interactions**.
• Select and view the video titled **0755: Disease Management**. (*Note:* Check the virtual clock to see whether enough time has elapsed. You can use the fast-forward feature to advance the time by 2-minute intervals if the video is not yet available. Then click on **Patient Care** and **Nurse-Client Interactions** to refresh the screen.)

18. While talking with his sitter, Harry George continues to voice the need for his own "medication." What technique does the sitter attempt to employ to manage this request?

Developing a Plan of Care for a Patient with Osteomyelitis

 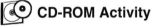 **Reading Assignment:** Care of the Patient with a Musculoskeletal Disorder
(Chapter 44)

Patient: Harry George, Room 401 (Disk 2)

Objectives:

1. Understand factors that affect pain management.
2. Identify nursing implications for the administration of narcotic analgesics.
3. Set priorities for the care of the patient with osteomyelitis.

Exercise 1

CD-ROM Activity

60 minutes

- Using the *Virtual Clinical Excursions—Medical-Surgical* CD (Disk 2), sign in to work at Pacific View Regional Hospital for Period of Care 2. (*Note:* If you are already in the virtual hospital from a previous exercise, click on **Leave the Floor** and then **Restart the Program** to get to the sign-in window.)
- From the Patient List, select Harry George (Room 401).
- Click on **Get Report** and read the Clinical Report.
- Click on **Go to Nurses' Station** and then on **401** to enter Harry George's room.
- Read the Initial Observation notes.
- Click on **Patient Care** and complete a head-to-toe assessment.

1. What are the two primary priorities for Harry George's care at this time?

2. What elements of the assessment or the Clinical Report did you use to make this decision?

3. How has pain interfered with Harry George's recovery?

4. Is Harry George's pain a new problem or one that has been ongoing? Give a rationale for your response.

5. What nonpharmacologic interventions can be used to attempt to increase Harry George's level of comfort?

→ • Click on **Patient Care** and then **Nurse-Client Interactions**.

• Select and view the video titled **1120: Wound Management**. (*Note:* Check the virtual clock to see whether enough time has elapsed. You can use the fast-forward feature to advance the time by 2-minute intervals if the video is not yet available. Then click on **Patient Care** and **Nurse-Client Interactions** to refresh the screen.)

6. What behaviors demonstrated by Harry George further support his report of pain and his level of anxiety?

• Now select and view the video titled **1125: Injury Prevention**. (*Note:* Check the virtual clock to see whether enough time has elapsed. You can use the fast-forward feature to advance the time by 2-minute intervals if the video is not yet available. Then click on **Patient Care** and **Nurse-Client Interactions** to refresh the screen.)

7. During the interaction with his sitter, Harry George continues to appear nervous. His movements reflect jitteriness, and his extremities are trembling. To what can these behaviors be attributed?

→ • Click on **MAR** and then on tab **401** to review Harry George's MAR.

8. The physician has prescribed chlordiazepoxide hydrochloride. Other than anxiety, what is an indication for the use of this medication?

9. Which of the following nursing implications are indicated with the administration of chlordiazepoxide hydrochloride? Select all that apply.

_____ Assess vital signs prior to administration.

_____ Increase ambulation immediately after administration.

_____ Administer cautiously in patients with liver impairments.

_____ Institute safety precautions in regard to ambulation.

_____ This medication may be used in patients who have recently ingested alcohol.

10. In addition to the chlordiazepoxide, what alternatives has the physician ordered to reduce Harry George's anxiety?

11. What factors will determine which of the medications should be given?

12. What medication has been ordered to manage Harry George's pain?

13. Does Harry George have any allergies that prevent him from being medicated with the drug prescribed? (*Hint:* Check his armband.)

14. Harry George's last dose of medication for pain was given at _____.

→ • Click on **Return to Room 401**. Then click on the **Drug** icon.
  • Review the information provided for the medication you identified in question 12.

15. What elements of Harry George's medical/social history should be taken into consideration when administering this drug?

16. Are there any special administration precautions that must be observed when giving this medication IV push?

17. Are there any special considerations that must be taken when administering this drug in conjunction with the other medications currently in use?

18. Identify any safety measures that should be observed after administration of this medication.

19. Is it time for Harry George to be medicated again for pain?

→ • Click on **Return to Room 401**. Then click on **Take Vital Signs**.

20. What are Harry George's vital signs?

    BP:

    SpO$_2$:

    T:

    HR:

    RR:

    Pain:

21. What impact has Harry George's pain had on his vital signs?

22. Are Harry George's vital signs within acceptable limits to administer the drug that has been ordered to manage his pain?

23. If Harry George is unable to take his prescribed medications, what action(s) would be appropriate?

LESSON **20**

Postoperative Assessment

Reading Assignment: Care of the Surgical Patient (Chapter 42)
Care of the Patient with a Musculoskeletal Disorder
(Chapter 44)

Patient: Clarence Hughes, Room 404 (Disk 2)

Objectives:

1. Define degenerative joint disease.
2. Identify the clinical signs and symptoms of degenerative joint disease.
3. Develop nursing diagnoses for the patient who has undergone joint replacement surgery.

Exercise 1

 Writing Activity

 15 minutes

1. Which of the following populations are at an increased risk for developing degenerative joint disease? Select all that apply.

   _____ Small-framed patients

   _____ Obese patients

   _____ Older patients

   _____ Patients employed in occupations with activities that place joints in stressful positions

   _____ Women of childbearing age

   _____ Patients with diabetes

2. Degenerative joint disease is a nonsystemic, noninflammatory disorder of the joints that results in bone and joint degeneration. What are some signs and symptoms of degenerative joint disease?

3. _____ and _____ are two other names for degenerative joint disease.

4. What are some management techniques for degenerative joint disease?

5. What is arthroscopy?

Exercise 2

 CD-ROM Activity

 45 minutes

- Using the *Virtual Clinical Excursions—Medical-Surgical* CD (Disk 2), sign in to work at Pacific View Regional Hospital for Period of Care 1. (*Note:* If you are already in the virtual hospital from a previous exercise, click on **Leave the Floor** and then **Restart the Program** to get to the sign-in window.)
- From the Patient List, select Clarence Hughes (Room 404).
- Click on **Get Report** and read the Clinical Report.
- Click on **Go to Nurses' Station** and then on **404** to enter Clarence Hughes' room.
- Read the Initial Observation notes.
- Click on **Chart** and then on **404** to view Clarence Hughes' chart.
- Click on the **History and Physical** tab and review the information given.

1. What signs and symptoms of degenerative joint disease has Clarence Hughes experienced?

2. What other methods of disease management did Clarence Hughes try prior to surgery?

- Click on **Return to Room 404**.
- Click on **Clinical Alerts** and read the information given.
- Now click on **Patient Care** and complete a head-to-toe assessment.

3. _____ Findings from Clarence Hughes' physical assessment warrant physician notification. (True or False)

4. What are the two most important priorities for care at this time?

5. Develop two individualized nursing diagnoses for this patient.

6. Why are these issues most important to the successful management of Clarence Hughes' care?

7. Are there any abnormal findings in the abdominal assessment?

→ • Click on **MAR** and then on tab **404** to review Clarence Hughes' record.

8. What medication options are available to manage Clarence Hughes' pain?

→ • Click on **Return to Room 404**.
  • Click on the **Drug** icon and review the pain medication(s) prescribed for Clarence Hughes.

9. Does Clarence Hughes have any contraindications for the pain medication(s) you identified in question 8?

10. What side effects can be anticipated with administration of the medication(s)?

11. Discuss any safety precautions that may need to be instituted with use of the medication(s).

12. Discuss any special monitoring that will be needed with the administration of the medication(s).

13. What regularly scheduled medication has been ordered to reduce the patient's constipation? What is the mechanism of action for this medication?

14. What prn medications have been ordered to reduce constipation? How do these medications work?

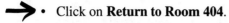 • Click on **Return to Room 404**.
- Click on **Chart** and then on **404** to view Clarence Hughes' chart.
- Click on the **Physician's Notes** tab.

15. What are the physician's plans concerning Clarence Hughes' discharge?

• Click on the **Consultations** tab.

16. What consultations have been ordered for Clarence Hughes? What is the purpose of these consultations?

• Click on the **Patient Education** tab.

17. What are Clarence Hughes' educational needs?

LESSON 21

Postoperative Complications

 Reading Assignment: Care of the Surgical Patient (Chapter 42)

Care of the Patient with a Respiratory Disorder (Chapter 49)

Patient: Clarence Hughes, Room 404 (Disk 2)

Objectives:

1. Identify potential postoperative complications.
2. Recognize clinical manifestations associated with the development of postoperative complications.
3. Review the management/treatment of a postoperative complication involving the respiratory system.

Exercise 1

 Writing Activity

15 minutes

1. List several potential postoperative complications.

2. The collapse of lung tissue, which results in the lack of adequate exchange of oxygen and

carbon dioxide, is known as _____.

179

Hint: Refer to pages 1688-1690 in your textbook for the next several questions.

3. What is a pulmonary embolism?

4. When you are assessing the patient for a pulmonary embolism, which of the following manifestations can be anticipated? Select all that apply.

_____ Dull and achy pain

_____ Pain often described as sharp

_____ Pain that radiates to the back and neck

_____ Nonradiating pain

_____ Dyspnea

_____ Reduced respiratory rate

_____ Increased respiratory rate

_____ Increased pain with inspiration

5. During the initial period after onset and subsequent diagnosis of pulmonary embolism, which of the following treatments can be anticipated? Select all that apply.

_____ Oxygen

_____ Oral anticoagulants

_____ Intramuscular antibiotics

_____ Intravenous anticoagulants

_____ Hydration

6. How is a pulmonary embolism managed?

7. What is the prognosis for a patient who develops a pulmonary embolism?

8. What is a ventilation perfusion scan?

Exercise 2

 CD-ROM Activity

 30 minutes

- Using the *Virtual Clinical Excursions—Medical-Surgical* CD (Disk 2), sign in to work at Pacific View Regional Hospital for Period of Care 2. (*Note:* If you are already in the virtual hospital from a previous exercise, click on **Leave the Floor** and then **Restart the Program** to get to the sign-in window.)
- From the Patient List, select Clarence Hughes (Room 404).
- Click on **Get Report** and read the Clinical Report.

1. Are there any abnormal observations in the change-of-shift report?

2. Review the vital signs recorded in the change-of-shift report. Are they normal?

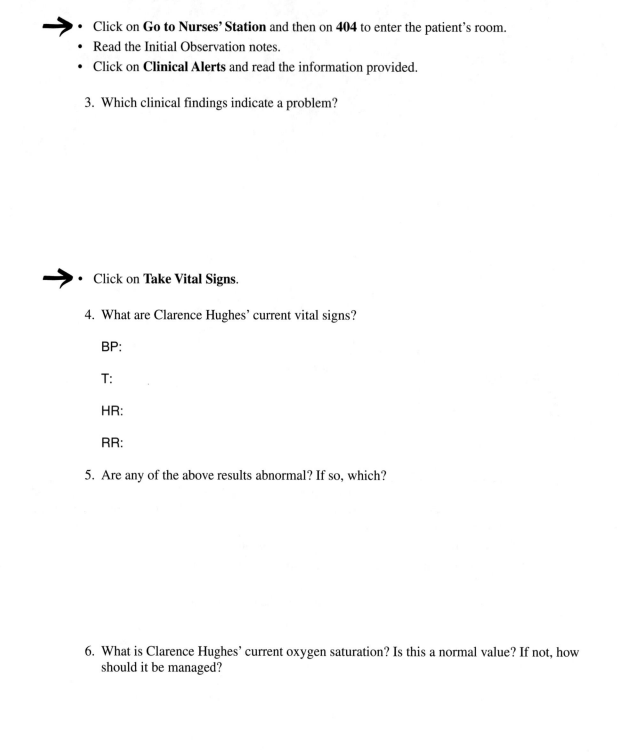

- Click on **Go to Nurses' Station** and then on **404** to enter the patient's room.
- Read the Initial Observation notes.
- Click on **Clinical Alerts** and read the information provided.

3. Which clinical findings indicate a problem?

- Click on **Take Vital Signs**.

4. What are Clarence Hughes' current vital signs?

BP:

T:

HR:

RR:

5. Are any of the above results abnormal? If so, which?

6. What is Clarence Hughes' current oxygen saturation? Is this a normal value? If not, how should it be managed?

• Click on **Patient Care** and then on **Nurse-Client Interactions**.
   • Select and view the video titled **1115: Interventions—Airway**. (*Note:* Check the virtual clock to see whether enough time has elapsed. You can use the fast-forward feature to advance the time by 2-minute intervals if the video is not yet available. Then click on **Patient Care** and **Nurse-Client Interactions** to refresh the screen.)

7. What behavioral cues being demonstrated by Clarence Hughes indicate a problem?

8. What should be the nurse's interventions (in priority order)?

 • Click on **Physical Assessment** and complete a head-to-toe assessment.

9. Are there any significant findings identified in the integumentary assessment?

10. Are there any significant findings identified in the respiratory assessment?

 • Click on **Chart** and then on **404** to view Clarence Hughes' chart.
   • Click on the **Physician's Orders** tab and review the orders listed for 1120 on Wednesday.

11. What tests and interventions has the physician ordered?

12. The degree of anxiety is often directly tied to the amount of _____
    hunger being experienced by the patient.

- Click on **Return to Room 404**.
- Click on **Patient Care** and then on **Nurse-Client Interactions**.
- Select and view the video titled **1135: Change in Patient Condition**. (*Note:* Check the virtual clock to see whether enough time has elapsed. You can use the fast-forward feature to advance the time by 2-minute intervals if the video is not yet available. Then click on **Patient Care** and **Nurse-Client Interactions** to refresh the screen.)

13. Now that the initial crisis has passed, what are the nurse's priorities concerning the family members?

Exercise 3

 CD-ROM Activity

 15 minutes

- Using the *Virtual Clinical Excursions—Medical-Surgical* CD (Disk 2), sign in to work at Pacific View Regional Hospital for Period of Care 3. (*Note:* If you are already in the virtual hospital from the previous exercise, click on **Leave the Floor** and then **Restart the Program** to get to the sign-in window.)
- From the Patient List, select Clarence Hughes (Room 404).
- Click on **Get Report** and read the Clinical Report.

1. Give the results for each of the tests listed below.

    Arterial blood gas:

    Chest x-ray:

    Ventilation perfusion scan:

    Doppler study:

• Click on **Go to Nurses' Station**.
 • Click on **404** to enter Clarence Hughes' room.
 • Read the Initial Observation notes.
 • Click on **Clinical Alerts** and review.

  2. What changes are noted in the patient's demeanor and clinical manifestations?

 • Click on **Take Vital Signs** and review the results.

  3. What is the significance of the increasing SpO_2 level?

 • Click on **Chart** and then on **404** to review Clarence Hughes' chart.
 • Click on the **Physician's Orders** tab and review the information given.

  4. What medication has been ordered to manage Clarence Hughes' condition? Describe the administration of this medication.

  5. What are the method of action and the purpose for the administration of this medication?

6. What is the classification of this medication?

7. During therapy with the medication identified in question 4, which of the following laboratory tests is most important to monitor?
   a. PTT
   b. Hgb
   c. Hct
   d. WBC
   e. ESR

LESSON **22** —————————————————————————

Care of the Patient with Pneumonia

 Reading Assignment: Care of the Patient with a Respiratory Disorder (Chapter 49)

Patient: Patricia Newman, Room 406 (Disk 2)

Objectives:

1. Define pneumonia.
2. Identify the potential causes of pneumonia.
3. Identify the populations at risk for pneumonia.
4. Discuss nursing care for the patient with pneumonia.

Exercise 1

 Writing Activity

30 minutes

   1. What is pneumonia?

   2. Infants and the _____ are most susceptible to pneumonia.

   3. What factors could make people more susceptible to pneumonia?

4. Which of the following may contribute to the development of pneumonia? Select all that apply.

   _____ Overuse of steroid medications

   _____ Infection

   _____ Hyperventilation

   _____ Inadequate ventilation

   _____ Aspiration

   _____ Poor nutritional habits

5. Match the columns below to show the correct order of pathologic occurrences associated with the development of pneumonia. (*Hint:* See page 1676 in your textbook.)

   Disease Process   **Order of Occurrence**

   _____ The respiratory tract develops inflammation   a. First
         and localized edema.
                                                                b. Second
   _____ The exchange of oxygen and carbon dioxide
         becomes increasingly reduced.   c. Third

   _____ Secretions begin to accumulate and are not able   d. Fourth
         to be moved by the cilia in the lungs.

   _____ Retained secretions become infected.

6. When caring for a patient diagnosed with pneumonia, which of the following nursing interventions are appropriate? Select all that apply.

   _____ Keep patient on complete bedrest.

   _____ Encourage deep breathing and coughing activities.

   _____ Initiate exercise training.

   _____ Provide patient education aimed at reducing the spread of infection.

   _____ Restrict protein intake.

   _____ Monitor vital signs and pulmonary status.

   _____ Provide information concerning the prescribed medication therapy.

   _____ Encourage fluid intake if not contraindicated by patient's coexisting conditions.

7. What is the typical prognosis for a patient with pneumonia?

 8. When assisting the patient with pneumonia to plan meals, which of the following dietary recommendations should be implemented? (*Hint:* See page 1678 in your textbook.)
   a. Three large balanced meals each day will be best to provide the needed nutrients.
   b. The diet should include at least 3000 calories per day.
   c. Protein and sodium are indicated.
   d. The diet should consist of at least 1500 calories each day.

9. What is the purpose of the above dietary intervention?

Exercise 2

 CD-ROM Activity

 45 minutes

- Using the *Virtual Clinical Excursions—Medical-Surgical* CD (Disk 2), sign in to work at Pacific View Regional Hospital for Period of Care 1. (*Note:* If you are already in the virtual hospital from a previous exercise, click on **Leave the Floor** and **Restart the Program** to get to the sign-in window.)
- From the Patient List, select Patricia Newman (Room 406).
- Click on **Get Report** and read the Clinical Report.
- Click on **Go to Nurses' Station**.
- Click on **Chart** and then **406** to view Patricia Newman's chart.
- Click on the **Emergency Department** tab and review the information given.

1. What were the findings of the Initial Assessment in the emergency department?

2. Discuss any abnormal findings in her respiratory system assessment.

3. Find the vital sign results on the ED record and discuss the significance of these findings.

4. What are the primary and secondary admitting diagnoses?

5. Listed below are laboratory tests ordered for Patricia Newman while in the emergency department. Match each laboratory test with its reason for being ordered.

Laboratory Test	**Reason It Was Ordered**
_____ Sputum gram stain	a. Ordered to provide information about the potential presence of infection and the body's response
_____ Arterial blood gases	b. Ordered to identify specific pathogens in a specimen
_____ Complete blood count	c. Ordered to identify the specific pathogens and determine which medications therapies will be most effective
_____ Culture and sensitivity	
_____ Erythrocyte sedimentation rate	d. Ordered to identify the presence and degree of inflammation in the body
	e. Ordered to definitely evaluate the oxygen levels in the body

6. What is the purpose of the x-ray ordered for this patient?

➡ • Click on **Return to Nurses' Station**.
   • Click on **406** and review the Initial Observation notes.

7. Discuss the significance of the oxygen saturation and the patient's removal of the nasal cannula.

8. _____ Patricia Newman's arterial blood gas results are within normal limits. (True or False)

➡ • Click on **Take Vital Signs** and review the results provided.

9. What are the patient's current vital signs, including oxygen saturation and pain level?

   BP:

   SpO$_2$:

   T:

   HR:

   RR:

   Pain:

10. What is the significance of these findings?

➡ • Click on **Patient Care** and complete a head-to-toe assessment.

11. What assessment findings support the admitting diagnosis of pneumonia?

➡ • Click on **MAR** and then on tab **406** to review the medications ordered for Patricia Newman.

12. The following drugs have been ordered to manage Patricia Newman's pneumonia. Match each drug with its correct classification.

Drug	Classification
_____ Acetaminophen	a. Antipyretic
_____ Cefotan	b. Antiinflammatory
_____ Ipratropium	c. Antibiotic
	d. Bronchodilator
	e. Corticosteroid

➡ • Click on **Return to Room 406**.
• Click on **Chart** and then on **406** to view Patricia Newman's chart.
• Click on the **Laboratory Reports** tab and review the information given.

13. Discuss the significance of the culture and sensitivity test results.

14. Review and discuss the findings of the complete blood count test.

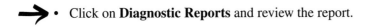 • Click on **Diagnostic Reports** and review the report.

15. Review the findings of the chest x-ray in relation to the diagnosis of pneumonia.

16. Which clinical manifestations will reflect positive impact of treatments?

LESSON **23** _____

Care of the Patient Experiencing Comorbid Conditions (Musculoskeletal and Respiratory)

_____

Reading Assignment: Care of the Patient with a Musculoskeletal Disorder
(Chapter 44)
Care of the Patient with a Cardiovascular or a Peripheral
Vascular Disorder (Chapter 48)
Care of the Patient with a Respiratory Disorder (Chapter 49)

Patient: Patricia Newman, Room 406 (Disk 2)

Objectives:

1. Identify significant findings in a patient's medical history.
2. Identify significant findings in a patient's social history.
3. Discuss the pathophysiology, risk factors, and management of hypertension.
4. Discuss the pathophysiology, risk factors, and management of osteoporosis.
5. Discuss the pathophysiology, risk factors, and management of emphysema.
6. Identify important issues in caring for the patient with comorbid conditions.

Exercise 1

 Writing Activity

 30 minutes

1. Hypertension occurs when blood pressure is sustained at systolic readings above

   _____ and/or diastolic readings greater than _____.

2. Which of the following risk factors are associated with hypertension? Select all that apply.

_____ Obesity

_____ Genetic factors

_____ Sedentary lifestyle

_____ Diabetes

_____ Asthma

_____ Increased sodium intake

_____ Excessive alcohol ingestion

3. List three medical management options for the treatment of hypertension.

4. What is emphysema?

5. What risk factors are associated with emphysema?

6. List several clinical manifestations of emphysema. (*Hint:* See page 1693 in your textbook.)

7. What are the management options for the patient with emphysema?

8. What is the usual prognosis for a patient diagnosed with emphysema?

9. Osteoporosis is a disease characterized by the reduction in _____.

10. Which of the following are at high risk for the development of osteoporosis? Select all that apply. (*Hint:* See page 1382 in your textbook.)

_____ Women

_____ Large-framed individuals

_____ Smokers

_____ Those with sedentary lifestyles

_____ People taking supplements to increase calcium intake

_____ Users of steroids

_____ Immobilized individuals

_____ Postmenopausal women

_____ African Americans

11. What areas of the body are most affected by osteoporosis?

12. List several clinical manifestations associated with osteoporosis.

13. When planning the care of a patient diagnosed with osteoporosis, which of the following may be included? Select all that apply.

    _____ Exercise

    _____ Restricted levels of activity

    _____ Increased calcium intake/supplements

    _____ Estrogen therapy

    _____ Reduced protein intake

14. To plan a diet high in calcium, which of the following should be included?
    a. Yellow vegetables
    b. Tomatoes
    c. Dates and legumes
    d. Green leafy vegetables

15. The coexistence of osteoporosis, emphysema, and hypertension presents what unique problems for Patricia Newman?

Exercise 2

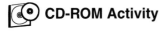 **CD-ROM Activity**

 45 minutes

- Using the *Virtual Clinical Excursions—Medical-Surgical* CD (Disk 2), sign in to work at Pacific View Regional Hospital for Period of Care 4. (*Note:* If you are already in the virtual hospital from a previous exercise, click on **Leave the Floor** and **Restart the Program** to get to the sign-in window.)
- Click on **Chart** and then **406** to view Patricia Newman's chart. (*Remember:* You are not able to visit patients or administer medications during Period of Care 4. You are able to review patients' records only.)
- Click on the **History and Physical** tab and review the information given.

1. What significant medical issues are in Patricia Newman's medical history?

2. Does the patient have any surgeries in her medical history?

3. Describe Patricia Newman's social history.

→ • Click on the **Nursing Admission** tab and review the information given.

4. What factors in Patricia Newman's history are related to a diagnosis of emphysema?

5. How is her recurring history of pneumonia related to her emphysema?

6. What factors in her history support a diagnosis of osteoporosis?

→ • Click on **Return to Nurses' Station**.
• Click on **MAR** and then on tab **406** to view the medications ordered for Patricia Newman.

7. What medications have been prescribed to manage Patricia Newman's hypertension?

8. Describe the mode of action for each of the medications you identified in question 7.

9. When you are planning care for the patient being treated with the above medications, which of the following laboratory tests must be monitored?
   a. Serum sodium levels
   b. Serum potassium levels
   c. Erythrocyte sedimentation rate
   d. Complete blood count results

10. What medications have been ordered to manage Patricia Newman's emphysema?

11. What medication has been prescribed to manage Patricia Newman's osteoporosis?

12. When you are administering the medication ordered to manage osteoporosis, which of the following nursing implications is indicated? Select all that apply.

   _____ Administer medication 15–30 minutes before eating.

   _____ Administer medication with juice to improve absorption.

   _____ Administer medication 30–60 minutes after eating.

   _____ Monitor blood pressure.

   _____ Administer with foods high in fiber.

Prioritizing Care for a Patient with a Pulmonary Disorder

—

📖 **Reading Assignment:** Care of the Patient with a Respiratory Disorder (Chapter 49)

Patient: Patricia Newman, Room 406 (Disk 2)

Objectives:

1. Identify the primary patient education goals for the patient experiencing a pulmonary disorder.
2. Discuss the appropriate service consultations for a patient experiencing a pulmonary disorder.
3. Determine the impact of personal/social factors in the patient's recovery period.
4. Develop priorities for the patient during hospitalization and in preparation for discharge.

Exercise 1

 Writing Activity

 30 minutes

1. Which of the following are characteristics associated with emphysema? Select all that apply.

   _____ Emphysema affects both men and women.

   _____ Emphysema symptoms typically begin to manifest while the patient is in the mid- to late 30s.

   _____ The disorder is characterized by changes in the alveolar walls and capillaries.

   _____ Disability often results in patients diagnosed with emphysema between ages 50 and 60 years.

   _____ Heredity may play a role in the development of emphysema.

2. When diagnostic tests are ordered to confirm the presence of emphysema, which of the following diagnostic tests should be anticipated? Select all that apply.

_____ Thoracentesis

_____ Arterial blood gases

_____ Complete blood cell count

_____ Chest x-ray

_____ Bronchoscopy

_____ Pulse oximetry

3. When caring for a patient diagnosed with emphysema, the nurse should anticipate which of the following results for a pulmonary function test?
   a. Reduced residual volume
   b. Reduced airway resistance
   c. Increased ventilatory response
   d. Increased residual volume

4. The complete blood cell count will reflect which of the following results in a patient diagnosed with emphysema?
   a. Reduced erythrocyte count
   b. Elevated erythrocyte count
   c. Elevated erythrocyte count and reduced hemoglobin
   d. Reduced erythrocyte count and elevated hemoglobin

5. In the patient who is experiencing emphysema, which of the following best reflects the anticipated pulmonary function tests?
   a. Increased PaO_2
   b. Decreased PaO_2
   c. Reduced residual volume
   d. Increased total lung capacity

6. Describe the disease process associated with emphysema.

7. Indicate whether each of the following statements is true or false.

   a. _____ An inherited form of emphysema is due to an oversecretion of a liver protein known as ATT.

   b. _____ Hypercapnia does not develop until the later stages of emphysema.

8. Discuss the use of exercise in the care and management of the patient diagnosed with emphysema.

9. _____ is an abnormal cardiac condition characterized by hypertrophy of the right ventricle of the heart due to hypertension of the pulmonary circulation.

10. The complete blood cell count will demonstrate which of the following characteristics in the patient with emphysema?
    a. The erythrocyte level will be within normal limits.
    b. The erythrocyte count will be elevated, and the hematocrit levels will be reduced.
    c. The erythrocytes, hematocrit, and hemoglobin values will be elevated.
    d. The erythrocyte count will be reduced, and the hematocrit and hemoglobin levels will be elevated.

Exercise 2

 CD-ROM Activity

 30 minutes

- Using the *Virtual Clinical Excursions—Medical-Surgical* CD (Disk 2), sign in to work at Pacific View Regional Hospital for Period of Care 3. (*Note:* If you are already in the virtual hospital from a previous exercise, click on **Leave the Floor** and **Restart the Program** to get to the sign-in window.)
- From the Patient List, select Patricia Newman (Room 406).
- Click on **Get Report** and read the Clinical Report.
- Click on **Go to Nurses' Station** and then on **406** to enter the patient's room.
- Read the Initial Observation notes.
- Click on **Patient Care** and then on **Nurse-Client Interactions**.
- Select and view the video titled **1500: Discharge Planning**. (*Note:* Check the virtual clock to see whether enough time has elapsed. You can use the fast-forward feature to advance the time by 2-minute intervals if the video is not yet available. Then click on **Patient Care** and **Nurse-Client Interactions** to refresh the screen.)

1. Discuss Patricia Newman's demeanor during the video interaction.

2. What appear to be the patient's biggest concerns during this interaction?

→ • Click on **Physical Assessment** and complete a head-to-toe assessment.

3. What evidence suggests that Patricia Newman's condition is improving?

4. Are there any assessment findings that have a potentially negative implication for Patricia Newman's discharge to home?

5. As you develop Patricia Newman's plan of care, which of the following are priorities at this time? Select all that apply.

_____ Dietary counseling

_____ Preparation for discharge

_____ Referrals for smoking cessation programs

_____ Requesting a consultation with physical therapy

_____ Requesting a consultation with social services

6. Develop three nursing diagnoses for Patricia Newman.

→ • Click on **Chart** and then on **406** to view Patricia Newman's chart.
• Click on the **Nursing Admission** tab and review the information given.

7. Identify Patricia Newman's social concerns.

8. Which of the following statements accurately reflects an aspect of the patient's needs?
   a. She has numerous friends and family members available to provide assistance.
   b. She appears self-sufficient and needs little outside help.
   c. She is somewhat socially isolated.
   d. Her significant other will be available as needed for assistance after discharge.

9. Discuss the implications of these social concerns on the nurse's plan of care for Patricia Newman.

→ • Click on the **Patient Education** tab and review the information given.

10. As Patricia Newman prepares to go home, which of the following are educational goals for her discharge? Select all that apply.

_____ Correct use of MDI and peak flow meter

_____ Understanding rationale for and performance of pursed-lip breathing and effective cough technique

_____ The need to be sedentary to avoid further complications

_____ Understanding of and compliance with prescribed medication therapy

_____ Compliance with progressive activity/exercise goals

11. Considering Patricia Newman's social and financial history, which of the goals may be a challenge for her to meet?

12. To assist Patricia Newman in complying with her discharge plans, consultations/referrals

    will be needed with _____ and

    _____ programs.

➤ • Click on the **Physician's Orders** tab.

13. What consultations have been ordered for Patricia Newman during this hospitalization?

LESSON **25** ———————————————————

Care of the Patient Experiencing Exacerbation of an Asthmatic Condition

—————————————————————————

📖 **Reading Assignment:** Care of the Patient with a Respiratory Disorder (Chapter 49)

Patient: Jacquline Catanazaro, Room 402 (Disk 2)

Objectives:

1. Define asthma.
2. Identify factors that contribute to an asthmatic episode.
3. Report assessment findings consistent with an exacerbation of asthma.
4. Discuss the impact of emotional distress on the respiratory system.

Exercise 1

 Writing Activity

 15 minutes

   1. What is asthma?

2. Which of the following events can trigger an asthmatic episode? Select all that apply.

_____ Hormone levels

_____ Mental and physical fatigue

_____ Emotional factors

_____ Environmental exposures

_____ Electrolyte imbalances

3. List the clinical manifestations of mild asthma.

4. Review the signs and symptoms associated with an acute asthmatic attack.

5. When an asthmatic condition is suspected, which of the following diagnostic tests will confirm a diagnosis? Select all that apply.

_____ Complete blood count

_____ Serum electrolyte levels

_____ Arterial blood gas

_____ Pulmonary function tests

_____ Sputum cultures

6. What is the prognosis for asthma?

7. Which of the following statements is correct concerning the impact of oxygen saturation levels on the body's functioning?
   a. Saturation rates of 95% to 100% are needed to replenish oxygen in the plasma.
   b. Saturation rates below 90% affect the ability of hemoglobin to feed oxygen to the plasma.
   c. Saturation levels below 70% are considered life-threatening.
   d. Saturation levels below 85% warrant contacting the physician.

Exercise 2

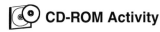 **CD-ROM Activity**

 45 minutes

- Using the *Virtual Clinical Excursions—Medical-Surgical* CD (Disk 2), sign in to work at Pacific View Regional Hospital for Period of Care 1. (*Note:* If you are already in the virtual hospital from a previous exercise, click on **Leave the Floor** and **Restart the Program** to get to the sign-in window.)
- From the Patient List, select Jacquline Catanazaro (Room 402).
- Click on **Get Report** and read the Clinical Report.
- Click on **Go to Nurses' Station**.
- Click on **Chart** and then on **402** to view Jacquline Catanazaro's chart.
- Click on the **Emergency Department** tab and review the information given.

1. Review the admitting vital signs. What is the significance of the findings?

2. What is the primary admitting diagnosis?

 • Click on **Return to Nurses' Station** and then on **402**.
- Read the Initial Observation notes.
- Click on **Take Vital Signs** and review the results provided.
- Click on **Clinical Alerts** and read the report.

3. Jacquline Catanazaro is demonstrating extreme agitation. What is the impact of these behaviors on her health status?

4. _____ When you are using the pulse oximeter, the probe should be placed over a pulsating vascular bed. (True or False)

5. When you are performing a pulse oximeter reading for the patient, which of the following sites is appropriate? Select all that apply.

_____ Ear lobe

_____ Bridge of the nose

_____ Tip of the nose

_____ Finger

_____ Toe

➤ • Click on **Patient Care** and then on **Nurse-Client Interactions**.
  • Select and view the video titled **0730: Intervention—Airway**. (*Note:* Check the virtual clock to see whether enough time has elapsed. You can use the fast-forward feature to advance the time by 2-minute intervals if the video is not yet available. Then click on **Patient Care** and **Nurse-Client Interactions** to refresh the screen.)

6. Jacquline Catanazaro is experiencing an acute asthma attack. What has been planned to manage the onset?

7. What will the arterial blood gases determine?

➤ • Click on **Physical Assessment** and complete a head-to-toe assessment.

8. What respiratory system findings in Jacquline Catanazaro's assessment are consistent with an exacerbation of asthma?

9. Are there any other significant system findings?

→ • Click on **Chart** and then on **402** to view Jacquline Catanazaro's chart.
   • Click on the **Physician's Orders** tab and note the admission orders for Monday at 1600.
   • Click on **Return to Room 402** and then on the **Drug** icon.
   • Review the information for the drugs that have been prescribed for Jacquline Catanazaro.

10. What are the doses and routes of administration for each medication ordered to manage Jacquline Catanazaro's respiratory condition?

    a. Beclomethasone:

    b. Albuterol:

    c. Ipratropium bromide:

11. Match each prescribed medication with its correct mode of action.

Medication	Mode of Action
_____ Beclomethasone	a. Relief of bronchospasms
_____ Albuterol	b. Reduction of bronchial inflammation
_____ Ipratropium bromide	c. Control of secretions

12. When providing patient education concerning the use of beclomethasone, the nurse should tell the patient that which of the following side effects may occur?
    a. Throat irritation
    b. Productive cough
    c. Increased pulmonary secretions
    d. Skin rash
    e. Activity intolerance

• Click on **Return to Room 402**.
- Click on **Chart** and then on **402**.
- Click on the **Physician's Orders** tab and review the orders for Monday at 1600.

13. What tests and/or assessments will be used to monitor Jacquline Catanazaro's respiratory status?

14. List several clinical manifestations that will indicate improvement in the patient's condition.

 • Click on **Return to Room 402**.
- Click on **Patient Care** and then on **Nurse-Client Interactions**.
- Select and view the video titled **0800: Managing Altered Perceptions**. (*Note:* Check the virtual clock to see whether enough time has elapsed. You can use the fast-forward feature to advance the time by 2-minute intervals if the video is not yet available. Then click on **Patient Care** and **Nurse-Client Interactions** to refresh the screen.)

15. What medication has been ordered for Jacquline Catanazaro?

16. What are the classification and mode of action for this medication?

Developing a Plan of Care for the Asthmatic Patient with Psychological Complications

---

∽ **Reading Assignment:** Care of the Patient with a Respiratory Disorder (Chapter 49)

Patient: Jacquline Catanazaro, Room 402 (Disk 2)

Objectives:

1. Evaluate the impact of the patient's social history on anticipated compliance after discharge.
2. Identify the elements to be incorporated into the teaching plan in preparation for discharge.
3. Develop nursing diagnoses for the patient experiencing coexisting psychological and physiological conditions.

Exercise 1

✐ Writing Activity

 15 minutes

1. _____ is a severe asthmatic attack that fails to respond to the normal treatment plan.

2. Extrinsic factors associated with an asthmatic attack include which of the following? Select all that apply.

   _____ Infection

   _____ Dust

   _____ Pollen

   _____ Exercise

   _____ Foods

3. Indicate whether each of the following statements is true or false.

   a. _____ Encouraging the patient experiencing an asthma attack to lean back will aid in breathing ability.

   b. _____ The death rate for asthma has been declining over the past 10 years because of the advances in pharmacologic therapies.

4. A complete blood cell count will reflect an elevation in which of the following in the patient experiencing an asthma attack?
   a. Eosinophils
   b. Platelets
   c. Red blood cells
   d. Monocytes

5. Which of the following is considered an acceptable range for a therapeutic level of theophylline?
   a. 35-45 mcg/mL
   b. Less than 4 mcg/mL
   c. 10-20 mcg/mL
   d. Greater than 50 mcg/mL

6. A _____ should be obtained to rule out a secondary infection.

7. Which of the following statements concerning asthma is true?
   a. Air tubes narrow as a result of swollen tissues and excessive mucus production.
   b. There is edema of respiratory mucosa and excessive mucous production, which obstructs airways.
   c. The walls of the alveoli are torn and cannot be repaired.
   d. The bronchioles are scarred and unable to expand.

8. Match each of the following drugs with its correct classification. (*Hint:* See page 1700 in your textbook.)

Drug	**Classification**
_____ Serevent	a. Corticosteroid
_____ Flovent	b. Long-acting beta receptor agonist
_____ Adrenalin	c. Short-acting beta receptor agonist
_____ Proventil	d. Bronchodilator

Exercise 2

 CD-ROM Activity

 45 minutes

- Using the *Virtual Clinical Excursions—Medical-Surgical* CD (Disk 2), sign in to work at Pacific View Regional Hospital for Period of Care 2. (*Note:* If you are already in the Virtual Hospital from a previous exercise, click on **Leave the Floor** and **Restart the Program** to get to the sign-in window.)
- From the Patient List, select Jacquline Catanazaro (Room 402).
- Click on **Get Report** and read the Clinical Report.

1. Describe the psychological behaviors documented in the two change-of-shift reports.

2. How do these psychological behaviors affect Jacquline Catanazaro's condition?

 - Click on **Go to Nurses' Station** and then on **402**.
- Read the Initial Observation notes.
- Click on **Take Vital Signs** and review the information given.
- Click on **Patient Care** and complete a head-to-toe assessment.
- Next, click on **Nurse-Client Interactions**.
- Select and view the video titled **1115: Assessment—Readiness to Learn**. (*Note:* Check the virtual clock to see whether enough time has elapsed. You can use the fast-forward feature to advance the time by 2-minute intervals if the video is not yet available. Then click on **Patient Care** and **Nurse-Client Interactions** to refresh the screen.)

3. What is the focus of the video interaction?

4. Do social supports appear to be available for Jacquline Catanazaro?

5. What are the priorities of care associated with Jacquline Catanazaro's psychosocial needs?

6. What are the priorities of care associated with Jacquline Catanazaro's physiological needs?

→ • Click on **Chart** and then on **402** to view Jacquline Catanazaro's chart.
  • Click on the **History and Physical** tab and review the information given.

7. List some significant issues identified in Jacquline Catanazaro's medical history.

8. List several significant issues identified in Jacquline Catanazaro's social history.

9. Describe the interrelationships among the medical and social elements in Jacquline Catanazaro's history.

10. What factors in Jacquline Catanazaro's medical history will significantly affect her discharge?

11. How does Jacquline Catanazaro's mental health affect her physical health?

→ • Click on the **Consultations** tab and review the information given.

12. Discuss the plan identified in the Psychiatric Consult report.

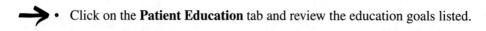 • Click on the **Patient Education** tab and review the education goals listed.

13. What are the educational goals identified?

14. Who should be included in the teaching plan for Jacquline Catanazaro?

15. Develop two nursing diagnoses for the patient at this point in her care.

LESSON 27 ———————————————————

Care and Treatment of the Patient with Complications of Cancer

───────────────────────────────────────

Reading Assignment: Care of the Patient with Cancer (Chapter 57)

Patient: Pablo Rodriguez, Room 405 (Disk 2)

Objectives:

1. Discuss complications associated with cancer.
2. Discuss the management of the patient experiencing dehydration secondary to chemotherapy.
3. Prioritize the problems of the patient experiencing complications of cancer.
4. Evaluate abnormal laboratory findings.

Exercise 1

 Writing Activity

 15 minutes

• Using the *Virtual Clinical Excursions—Medical-Surgical* CD (Disk 2), sign in to work at Pacific View Regional Hospital for Period of Care 2. (*Note:* If you are already in the virtual hospital from a previous exercise, click on **Leave the Floor** and then **Restart the Program** to get to the sign-in window.)
• From the Patient List, select Pablo Rodriguez (Room 405).
• Click on **Get Report** and read the Clinical Report.
• Click on **Go to Nurses' Station**.
• Click on **Chart** and then **405** to view Pablo Rodriguez's chart.
• Click on **Emergency Department** and review the information given.

  1. What are the four priorities identified in the change-of-shift report?

2. Why was Pablo Rodriguez admitted to the hospital?

3. What has caused this condition?

4. What findings support this diagnosis?

5. How was his condition initially managed in the emergency department?

6. What types of interventions (nursing and medical) may be implemented to manage his care?

7. What should be monitored to determine the degree of dehydration?

8. What are the primary goals for this hospitalization?

 • Click on the **History and Physical** tab and read the report.

9. List the impressions identified in the History and Physical.

Exercise 2

 CD-ROM Activity

 30 minutes

- Using the *Virtual Clinical Excursions—Medical-Surgical* CD (Disk 2), sign in to work at Pacific View Regional Hospital for Period of Care 2. (*Note:* If you are already in the virtual hospital from a previous exercise, click on **Leave the Floor** and **Restart the Program** to get to the sign-in window.)
- From the Patient List, select Pablo Rodriguez (Room 405).
- Click on **Go to Nurses' Station**.
- Click on **405** to enter Pablo Rodriguez's room.
- Read the Initial Observation notes.
- Click on **Take Vital Signs** and then on **Clinical Alerts** and review the information given.
- Click on **Patient Care** and complete a head-to-toe assessment.

1. What current assessment findings support the diagnosis of dehydration?

→ • Click on **Chart** and then on **405** to view Pablo Rodriguez's chart.
  • Click on **Physician's Orders** and review the orders since Tuesday at 2300.

2. Which medications have been ordered to manage Pablo Rodriguez's nausea?

→ • Click on **Return to Room 405** and then on the **Drug** icon.
  • Review the medications you identified in the previous question.

3. To what drug classification does ondansetron hydrochloride belong?

4. What side effects of ondansetron could be problematic, considering Pablo Rodriguez's health concerns?

5. What is metoclopramide's mechanism of action?

→ • Click on **Return to Room 405**.
  • Once again, click on **Chart** and then on **405**.
  • This time, click on **Laboratory Reports** and review the report given.

6. Review and discuss any significant findings in the CBC results.

7. What signs and symptoms may be attributed to the CBC results?

8. Are there any significant findings in the electrolyte profile?

9. Identify two nursing diagnoses related to Pablo Rodriguez's primary admitting diagnosis.

Exercise 3

 CD-ROM Activity

 30 minutes

- Using the *Virtual Clinical Excursions—Medical-Surgical* CD (Disk 2), sign in to work at Pacific View Regional Hospital for Period of Care 2. (*Note:* If you are already in the virtual hospital from a previous exercise, click on **Leave the Floor** and then **Restart the Program** to get to the sign-in window.)
- From the Patient List, select Pablo Rodriguez (Room 405).
- Click on **Get Report** and read the Clinical Report.
- Click on **Go to Nurses' Station** and then on **405** to enter Pablo Rodriguez's room.
- Click on **Take Vital Signs** and review the information given.

1. How does Pablo Rodriguez rate his pain?

→ • Click on **MAR** and then on tab **405** to review the medications ordered for Pablo Rodriguez.

2. What medications have been ordered to manage Pablo Rodriguez's pain?

3. What is the advantage of this type of dosing?

4. List some opioids that may be prescribed to manage the pain associated with advanced cancer.

5. What side effects are associated with opioid administration?

6. List several nonopioid medications that can be administered to reduce mild to moderate pain associated with cancer.

7. Discuss medication scheduling techniques that effectively manage pain.

8. As previously stated, Pablo Rodriguez has been experiencing anxiety. Discuss the relationship between pain and anxiety.

9. In addition to medication therapy, what other interventions may be used to manage pain?

10. What factors may influence a patient's perception of and/or reaction to pain?

 • Click on **Return to Room 405**.
 • Click on **Patient Care** and then on **Nurse-Client Interactions**.
 • Select and view the video titled **1130: Family Interaction**. (*Note:* Check the virtual clock to see whether enough time has elapsed. You can use the fast-forward feature to advance the time by 2-minute intervals if the video is not yet available. Then click on **Patient Care** and **Nurse-Client Interactions** to refresh the screen.)

11. What is the underlying message Pablo Rodriguez is attempting to communicate to his daughter?
    a. He is too tired to attend her wedding.
    b. The enema has made him feel better.
    c. He is ready to give in to the disease and die.
    d. The enema has caused him pain.

12. Does the response by Pablo Rodriguez's daughter indicate a readiness to accept her father's condition?

13. _____ Pablo Rodriguez will be allowed to make the decision to forego further treatment without the approval of his immediate family. (True or False)

14. Identify referrals that may be beneficial for Pablo Rodriguez and his family at this time.

LESSON 28

Care and Treatment of the Patient with Cancer

Reading Assignment: Care of the Patient with Cancer (Chapter 57)

Patient: Pablo Rodriguez, Room 405 (Disk 2)

Objectives:

1. Identify the physiological changes associated with the diagnosis of cancer.
2. List risk factors for the development of cancer.
3. Identify the tests that may be used to diagnose cancer.
4. Define metastasis.

Exercise 1

 Writing Activity

 30 minutes

1. Which of the following foods have been shown to reduce the risk for cancer? Select all that apply.

   _____ Broccoli

   _____ Lettuce

   _____ Bananas

   _____ Carrots

   _____ Grapefruit

   _____ Tomatoes

2. Adding at least _____ servings of fruits and vegetables per day has been shown to reduce the risk for cancer.

3. _____ The risk for the development of lung cancer is similar among users of smokeless tobacco and cigarette smokers. (True or False)

229

4. Match each diagnostic test with its correct description. (*Hint:* See page 2067 in your textbook.)

Diagnostic Test	**Description**
_____ Computed tomography	a. The use of noninvasive, high-frequency sound waves to examine external body structures.
_____ Radioisotope studies	
_____ Ultrasound testing	b. A computer is employed to process radio-frequency energy waves to assess spinal lesions, as well as cardiovascular and soft tissue abnormalities.
_____ Magnetic resonance imaging	
	c. The use or radiographs and computed scanning to provide images of structures at differing angles.
	d. A substance is injected or ingested; then the uptake is evaluated to identify areas of concern.

5. Which of the following characteristics are associated with benign growths? Select all that apply.

_____ Rapid growth

_____ Smooth and well-defined

_____ Immobile when palpated

_____ Often recurs after removal

_____ Crowds normal tissue

_____ Remains localized

 6. Match each diagnostic laboratory test with the type of cancer it is used to detect. (*Hint:* See page 2068 in your textbook.)

Diagnostic Test	**Type of Cancer Detected**
_____ Serum calcitonin levels	a. Thyroid, breast, and oat (small) cell cancer in the lung
_____ Carcinoembryonic antigen	
	b. Gynecologic and pancreatic cancers
_____ PSA	
	c. Prostate cancer
_____ CA-125	
	d. Colorectal cancer

7. The complete blood cell profile of a patient diagnosed with cancer shows a reduction in the number of circulating platelets. Which of the following terms is used to describe this condition?
   a. Leukopenia
   b. Thrombocytopenia
   c. Anemia
   d. Neutropenia

8. Discuss the use of radiation treatments to manage cancer.

9. What is the mode of action for chemotherapy drugs?

10. Sometimes cancer is described as metastatic. What does this mean?

11. How does metastasis occur?

12. What diagnostic tools may be used to identify cancer? (*Hint:* See pages 2066-2068 in your textbook.)

13. Use of the immune system to counteract the destruction of cancer cells is known as

_____. _____ may be used to remove a tumor, lesion, and surrounding malignant tissue.

14. Indicate whether each of the following statements is true or false.

a. _____ Alopecia in patients undergoing chemotherapy results from damage to the hair follicle.

b. _____ Alopecia is permanent.

c. _____ Hair that regrows may be of a different color and/or texture than original hair.

15. List and discuss the complications involving the gastrointestinal system associated with the administration of chemotherapy.

16. Why is the patient with cancer at risk for developing nutritional problems?

17. For what nutritional disturbances is the patient with cancer at risk?

Exercise 2

 CD-ROM Activity

 30 minutes

- Using the *Virtual Clinical Excursions—Medical-Surgical* CD (Disk 2), sign in to work at Pacific View Regional Hospital for Period of Care 4. (*Note:* If you are already in the virtual hospital from a previous exercise, click on **Leave the Floor** and **Restart the Program** to get to the sign-in window.)
- Click on **Chart** and then **405** to view Pablo Rodriguez's chart. (*Remember:* You are not able to visit patients or administer medications during Period of Care 4. You are able to review patients' records only.)
- Click on **Nursing Admission** and review the information given.

1. What is Pablo Rodriguez's medical diagnosis?

2. According to the Nursing Admission, how does the patient describe his prognosis?

3. When was Pablo Rodriguez diagnosed with lung cancer?

→ • Click on **History and Physical** and review the reports.

4. How has Pablo Rodriguez's cancer been treated?

5. Does he have any family history of cancer?

6. Does his social history contain any risk factors for his diagnosis of lung cancer?

7. What psychosocial changes have resulted in his life because of the cancer?

8. Discuss the physical changes that have taken place as a result of Pablo Rodriguez's cancer.

9. Discuss Pablo Rodriguez's emotional readiness for death.

10. What emotional concerns have been voiced by the patient?

11. What therapeutic behaviors by the nurse are essential at this time?

12. What factors may put Pablo Rodriguez at risk for infection?

13. In addition to the nausea and vomiting, is Pablo Rodriguez suffering from any other complications of the gastrointestinal system?

14. Has Pablo Rodriguez experienced any nutritional disturbances during his illness?

LESSON **29**

Assessment of the Patient with Gastrointestinal Complications

Reading Assignment: Care of the Patient with a Gastrointestinal Disorder (Chapter 45)

Patient: Piya Jordan, Room 403 (Disk 2)

Objectives:

1. Identify clinical manifestations and causes of intestinal obstructions.
2. Develop nursing diagnoses appropriate for the patient experiencing an intestinal obstruction.
3. Explain operative measures used in cases of intestinal obstruction.
4. Identify common gastrointestinal disorders.
5. Identify tests used in the diagnosis of gastrointestinal disorders.
6. List medications used in the management of gastrointestinal disorders.

Exercise 1

Writing Activity

 15 minutes

1. Describe the two types of intestinal obstructions.

   a. Mechanical obstruction:

   b. Nonmechanical obstruction:

2. The signs and symptoms associated with a bowel obstruction will be determined by the

_____ and _____ of _____.

3. Early manifestations of an intestinal obstruction include which of the following? Select all that apply.

_____ Loud bowel sounds

_____ High-pitched bowel sounds

_____ Vomiting

_____ Constipation

_____ Absence of bowel sounds

_____ Frequent bowel sounds

_____ Abdominal pain

4. Identify several causes of mechanical intestinal obstructions. (*Hint:* See page 1482 in your textbook.)

5. Which of the following are causes associated with non-mechanical intestinal obstructions? Select all that apply.

_____ Complications from surgery

_____ Bowel tumors

_____ Electrolyte abnormalities

_____ Thoracic spinal trauma

_____ Lumbar spinal trauma

_____ Emboli or atherosclerosis of the mesenteric arteries

_____ Impacted feces

6. _____ Paralytic ileus is the most common type of nonmechanical intestinal obstruction. (True or False)

7. Which of the following symptoms, if present, can be associated with a paralytic ileus? Select all that apply.

_____ Increased abdominal girth

_____ Distention

_____ Urinary frequency

_____ Elevated white blood cell count

_____ Vomiting

8. Which of the following interventions are done to reduce the risk for developing a paralytic ileus? Select all that apply.

_____ Abdominal assessment

_____ IV therapy

_____ Maintenance of NG tube

_____ Increase in patient activity

_____ Deep breathing exercises

Exercise 2

Writing Activity

30 minutes

1. Match each diagnostic test with its correct description.

Diagnostic Test

_____ Upper gastrointestinal study

_____ Tube gastric analysis

_____ Esophagogastroduodenoscopy

_____ Lower GI endoscopy

_____ Bernstein test

Description

a. Aspiration and review of stomach contents to determine acid production

b. Radiographs of the lower esophagus, stomach, and duodenum using barium sulfate at a contrast medium

c. Visualization of the upper GI tract by a flexible scope

d. An acid-perfusion test using hydrochloric acid

e. Assessment of the lower GI tract with a scope

2. What is a KUB?

3. When providing education to a patient diagnosed with GERD, which of the following will need to be included in the teaching session? Select all that apply.

_____ Eat a low-fat, low-protein diet

_____ Avoid eating 4 to 6 hours before bedtime

_____ Remain upright for 1 to 2 hours after meals

_____ Avoid eating in bed

_____ Eat 4 to 6 small meals per day

_____ Reduce caffeine intake

4. Match each gastrointestinal disorder with its correct description.

Gastrointestinal Disorder	Description
_____ GERD	a. The presence of pouchlike herniations through the muscular layers of the colon
_____ Candidiasis	b. Characterized by inflammation of segments of the GI tract, resulting in a cobblestone-like appearance of the mucosa
_____ Gastritis	
_____ Irritable bowel syndrome	c. Episodic bowel dysfunction characterized by intestinal pain, disturbed defecation, or abdominal distention
_____ Ulcerative colitis	
_____ Crohn's disease	d. The formation of tiny abscesses on mucosa and submucosa of the colon, producing drainage and sloughing of the mucosa and subsequent ulcerations
_____ Diverticulosis	
	e. The backward flow of stomach acid into the esophagus
	f. A fungal infection presenting as white patches on the mucous membranes
	g. Inflammation of the lining of the stomach

5. Match each gastrointestinal medication with its correct classification.

   Medication   **Classification**

   _____ Maalox   a. Proton pump inhibitor

   _____ Pepcid   b. Antacid

   _____ Prevacid   c. Antisecretory and cytoprotective agent

   _____ Carafate   d. Mucosal healing agent

   _____ Cytotec   e. Histamine H_2 receptor blocker

6. Which of the following alternative therapies may provide relief for excessive flatulence? Select all that apply.

   _____ Comfrey

   _____ Queen Anne's lace seeds

   _____ Anise

   _____ Chaparral

   _____ Peppermint oil

   _____ Spearmint extract

7. Gastrointestinal disorders may be more prevalent in certain ethnic groups. Which of the following ethnic groups has a higher incidence of inflammatory bowel disease?
   a. Caucasian
   b. African-American
   c. Asian-American
   d. Americans of Middle Eastern descent

8. The increased incidence of gastritis in older adults can be attributed to the decreased secretion of _____.

9. What is a colectomy? What is a colostomy?

Exercise 3

 CD-ROM Activity

 15 minutes

- Using the *Virtual Clinical Excursions—Medical-Surgical* CD (Disk 2), sign in to work at Pacific View Regional Hospital for Period of Care 1. (*Note:* If you are already in the virtual hospital from a previous exercise, click on **Leave the Floor** and then **Restart the Program** to get to the sign-in window.)
- From the Patient List, select Piya Jordan (Room 403).
- Click on **Get Report** and read the Clinical Report.
- Click on **Go to Nurse's Station**.
- Click on **Chart** and then on **403** to view Piya Jordan's chart.
- Click on the **Emergency Department** tab and review the information given.

1. What are Piya Jordan's primary complaints upon arrival to the emergency department?

2. What are Piya Jordan's vital signs at admission?

   HR:

   T:

   RR:

   BP:

3. Piya Jordan's hypotension can most likely be attributed to which of the following?
   a. The presence of infection
   b. An elevation in blood glucose values
   c. Hypokalemia
   d. Dehydration

4. What diagnostic tests were ordered in the emergency department?

5. According to the ED Physician's Progress Notes, what are the abnormal findings on the physical assessment that support a potential bowel obstruction?

6. What are the treatment goals of the care for a patient experiencing an intestinal obstruction?

7. Initial management of the patient's condition included the placement of an NG tube. The NG tube can serve a variety of functions. Match each function with its correct description.

Function	Description
_____ Decompression	a. Irrigation of the stomach, used in cases of active bleeding, poisoning, or gastric dilation
_____ Feeding	b. Removal of secretions and gases from the GI tract
_____ Compression	c. Internal application of pressure by means of an inflated balloon to prevent internal GI hemorrhage
_____ Lavage	d. Instillation of liquid supplements into the stomach

8. Piya Jordan has had the NG tube inserted for _____.

→ • Click on **Return to Nurses' Station** and then on **403** to go to Piya Jordan's room.
   • Review the Initial Observation notes.

9. According to the Initial Observations, blood is being administered to Piya Jordan. What laboratory results will necessitate close observation to determine the effectiveness of this intervention?

10. What will the nurse need to monitor concerning the blood transfusion?

11. Piya Jordan has remained NPO since the surgery. What information will the nurse need to monitor to ensure she is adequately hydrated?

Colorectal Cancer and Care of the Patient After Gastrointestinal Surgery

/⚬⚬⚬ **Reading Assignment:** Care of the Surgical Patient (Chapter 42)
Care of the Patient with a Gastrointestinal Disorder (Chapter 45)

Patient: Piya Jordan, Room 403 (Disk 2)

Objectives:

1. Identify risk factors associated with the development of colorectal cancer.
2. List the warning signs and symptoms associated with a diagnosis of colorectal cancer.
3. Identify the assessment priorities for the postoperative patient.
4. Discuss the safe use of narcotics administered in the postoperative period.
5. Discuss the potential for postoperative complications.

Exercise 1

 Writing Activity

 15 minutes

1. Indicate whether each of the following statements is true or false.

   a. _____ Cancer of the colon and rectum is the second leading cause of cancer in the United States.

   b. _____ In the early stages, colorectal cancer is often asymptomatic.

2. Match each location for colorectal cancer with its frequency of incidence. (*Hint:* See page 1484 in your textbook.)

Location of Cancer	Frequency of Incidence
_____ Transverse splenic flexure, hepatic flexure, and descending colon	a. 45%
_____ Sigmoid and rectal	b. 25%
_____ Cecum and descending colon	c. 30%

3. The incidence of colorectal cancer is associated with which of the following? Select all that apply.

   _____ Ulcerative colitis

   _____ Peritonitis

   _____ Diverticulosis

   _____ Elevated bacterial counts in the colon

   _____ Vegan diets

   _____ High dietary fat intake

   _____ Dietary intake high in cruciferous vegetables

4. A patient at age 36 with a family history of colon cancer should follow which of the following recommendations for screening?
   a. Begin colonoscopy screening after age 50.
   b. Participate in a baseline colonoscopy prior to age 50.
   c. An initial colonoscopy should be performed prior to age 40 and repeated every 5 years.
   d. No special screening recommendations are needed.

5. Which of the following symptoms are associated with the later stages of colorectal cancer? Select all that apply.

   _____ Constipation

   _____ Diarrhea

   _____ Abdominal pain

   _____ Anemia

   _____ Weakness

   _____ Emaciation

6. The incidence of colorectal cancer increases in persons over age _____.

7. The 5-year survival rate for early localized colorectal cancer is _____%; for cancer that has spread to adjacent organs and lymph nodes, it is _____%.

8. _____ refers to weakness and emaciation associated with general ill health and malnutrition.

9. What details should be included in the assessment of a surgical incision?

Exercise 2

 CD-ROM Activity

 30 minutes

- Using the *Virtual Clinical Excursions—Medical-Surgical* CD (Disk 2), sign in to work at Pacific View Regional Hospital for Period of Care 1. (*Note:* If you are already in the virtual hospital from a previous exercise, click on **Leave the Floor** and **Restart the Program** to get to the sign-in window.)
- From the Patient List, select Piya Jordan (Room 403).
- Click on **Get Report** and read the Clinical Report.
- Click on **Go to Nurses' Station** and then on the **Drug** icon. Find the entry for meperidine and review.

1. Based on your review of the shift report, which care factors appear to be of high priority?

2. The assessment findings of which of the patient's body systems demonstrate the potential for developing postoperative complications?
   a. Respiratory system
   b. Renal system
   c. Integumentary system
   d. Reproductive system

- Click on **Return to Nurses' Station**.
- Click on **403** and read the Initial Observation notes.
- Click on **Take Vital Signs** and then on **Clinical Alerts** and review the information given.
- Click on **Patient Care** and complete a head-to-toe assessment.

3. Discuss the proper assessment of bowel sounds for this patient.

4. What is the purpose of the Jackson-Pratt drain? How long will it need to be in place for Piya Jordan?

5. When providing care for Piya Jordan, what should the nurse monitor and record regarding the NG tube?

6. Piya Jordan has a reduced aeration to the left lower lobe. What interventions can promote improved aeration and a reduction in potential complications?

→ • Click on **Chart** and then on **403** to view Piya Jordan's chart.
   • Click on the **Nurse's Notes** tab and review the information given.

7. According to the Wednesday 0630 Nurse's Notes, Piya Jordan's meperidine PCA was dis-
continued because of suspicions of toxicity. Which of the following clinical manifestations
are associated with meperidine toxicity? Select all that apply.

_____   Respiratory depression

_____   Systolic hypertension

_____   Clammy skin

_____   Cyanosis

_____   Stupor

_____   Coma

_____   Diarrhea

8. In the event that pharmacologic intervention is needed to treat meperidine toxicity, which of
the following medications may be administered?
   a. Compazine
   b. Phenergan
   c. Morphine
   d. Narcan
   e. Famotidine

9. Which of the following conditions may increase a patient's risk for meperidine toxicity?
Select all that apply.

_____   Advancing age

_____   Diabetes

_____   Cardiovascular disorders

_____   Renal impairments

_____   Hypertension

→ • Click on **Return to Room 403**.
  • Click on **Physical Assessment** and complete a head-to-toe assessment.

10. Which of the following assessment findings for Piya Jordan are in accordance with the suspected meperidine toxicity? Select all that apply.

_____   Glasgow Coma Scale results

_____   Confusion

_____   Temperature 99.9

_____   Respiratory rate 23

_____   Slurred, slowed speech

_____   Restless

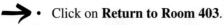 • Click on **Return to Room 403**.

- Click on **Patient Care** and then on **Nurse-Client Interactions**.

- Select and view the video titled **0735: Pain—Adverse Drug Event**. (*Note:* Check the virtual clock to see whether enough time has elapsed. You can use the fast-forward feature to advance the time by 2-minute intervals if the video is not yet available. Then click on **Patient Care** and **Nurse-Client Interactions** to refresh the screen.)

11. What problems were encountered during the previous evening with regard to the use of the PCA pump?

12. What patient/family concerns during the video indicate the need for education?

13. What issues does the nurse need to address with Piya Jordan's daughter in particular?

Exercise 3

 CD-ROM Activity

 30 minutes

- Using the *Virtual Clinical Excursions—Medical-Surgical* CD (Disk 2), sign in to work at Pacific View Regional Hospital for Period of Care 3. (*Note:* If you are already in the virtual hospital from a previous exercise, click on **Leave the Floor** and then **Restart the Program** to get to the sign-in window.)
- From the Patient List, select Piya Jordan (Room 403).
- Click on **Get Report** and read the Clinical Report.
- Click on **Go to Nurses' Station** and then on **403** to enter the patient's room.
- Read the Initial Observation notes.

1. Have there been any changes in mental status since Period of Care 1?

2. What changes have been made to the type and/or administration of Piya Jordan's pain medication?

3. How does Piya Jordan rate her pain at this time?

→ - Click on **Chart** and then on **403** to view Piya Jordan's chart.
- Click on **Surgical Reports** and review the reports.

4. What type of surgery was planned for Piya Jordan? What surgical procedure was actually completed?

5. Which of the following are the most common complications associated with the surgery performed on Piya Jordan? Select all that apply.

_____ Hemorrhage

_____ Infection

_____ Blood loss

_____ Pneumonia

_____ Wound dehiscence

_____ Blood clots

_____ Paralytic ileus

6. What is Piya Jordan's postoperative diagnosis?

➜ • Click on **Physician's Orders** and review the information given.

7. What medications and/or interventions have been ordered to assess and reduce the patient's postoperative risk of infection?

8. Which of the following assessments will provide information to determine the presence of an infection? Select all that apply.

_____ Vital signs

_____ Appearance of urine in Foley catheter bag

_____ Abdominal incision

_____ Lung fields

_____ Patency of Jackson-Pratt drain

→ • Click on **Return to Room 403**.
  • Click on **Take Vital Signs** and review the information given.
  • Click on **Patient Care** and perform a head-to-toe assessment.

9. Does Piya Jordan demonstrate any symptoms associated with a potential infection?

10. What interventions have been ordered to reduce the patient's risk for pulmonary complications?